Data Analysis with Competing Risks and Intermediate States

Chapman & Hall/CRC Biostatistics Series

Published Titles

Chapman & Hall/CRC Biostatistics Series

Data Analysis with Competing Risks and Intermediate States

Ronald B. Geskus

Academic Medical Center

and

Public Health Service of Amsterdam

Amsterdam, The Netherlands

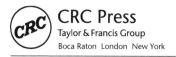

CRC Press
Taylor & Francis Group
Boca Raton London New York

CRC Press is an imprint of the
Taylor & Francis Group, an **informa** business
A CHAPMAN & HALL BOOK

CRC Press
Taylor & Francis Group
6000 Broken Sound Parkway NW, Suite 300
Boca Raton, FL 33487-2742

© 2016 by Taylor & Francis Group, LLC
CRC Press is an imprint of Taylor & Francis Group, an Informa business

No claim to original U.S. Government works

ISBN 13: 978-1-4665-7035-1 (hbk)

Visit the Taylor & Francis Web site at
http://www.taylorandfrancis.com

and the CRC Press Web site at
http://www.crcpress.com

To life

Contents

Preface

In the end we all die. More interesting than the death event itself is the time component: at what age does one die and what characteristics make some individuals die earlier than others? Survival analysis provides the set of tools that help answer the question of which factors influence the time until the occurrence of some event, which is not restricted to be death.

In the end we all die, but not all from the same cause. Information on the spectrum of causes of death has added value. Figure 1 shows the number of individuals that died of different causes in the twentieth century. The smallest

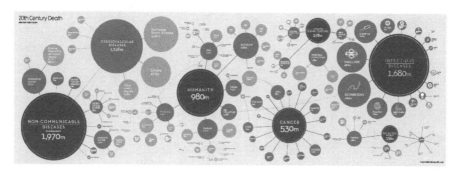

FIGURE 1
All causes of death in the 20th century.

subgroups may not be readable (have a look at the website if you want to read them[1]), but it is seen that the most frequent category is made up of the non-communicable diseases, within which cardiovascular diseases form the largest subgroup. The causes of death are competing: if one occurs, the others do not. Again, including the time component has added value. Some causes, like measles, tend to occur at a young age, whereas others, like prostate cancer, almost exclusively occur in older men. Measles mortality prevents prostate cancer from occurring, but if mortality due to measles is reduced, mortality due to prostate cancer, at a later age, may rise. A competing risks model extends the classical survival setting by considering a collection of mutually

---

[1]The figure was downloaded on September 1st, 2013 from the website
http://www.informationisbeautiful.net/visualizations/20th-century-death.
Author: David McCandless.

exclusive potential event types. Different causes of death are the classical example, but any set of event types can be considered.

The issues that come up when competing risks are present have often been ignored, even in top (medical) journals [61]. But the situation is changing rapidly. In the last decade, several papers have been published that explain when and why a standard time-to-event approach fails to provide the correct answer. Still, confusion remains with respect to the quantities that can be estimated and their interpretation. Fortunately, once the concepts are understood and the appropriate type of analysis has been chosen, techniques of estimation are not much different from the ones used in classical survival analysis with only one event type.

In the end we all die, but not all for the same reason nor with the same life histories. Even if two individuals die at the same age and of the same cause, their life courses have been different. Between birth and death, intermediate events occur that influence one's life course. The are several ways to model the occurrence of such events and their effect on later ones. One approach is via a multi-state model, in which events are seen as transitions from one state to another. Death may be the final one, but the process under investigation may terminate earlier. Under the frequently assumed Markov property, a multi-state model can be seen as a sequence of competing risks models.

Multi-state models can give a more detailed description of a disease process. Only few articles have explained the use of multi-state models to non-statisticians. Although the range of modeling choices and possible assumptions is larger than in a competing risks setting, there is little additional complexity with respect to interpretation. Also, some of the estimation techniques are a direct extension of those from the competing risks setting such that the same software can be used. Other computations are more complex and require software that has been written specifically for such models.

This book is divided into five chapters and an epilogue. The first chapter introduces the main concepts, with emphasis on the competing risks setting. For a number of examples that will be used throughout the book, we formulate the type of questions that may be of interest and define the corresponding estimands. We explain when the data at hand can be used to answer these questions. We also give an overview of the main definitions and techniques from classical survival analysis that are used and extended in later chapters. In Chapters 2 and 3 we more formally define the concepts that play a role in competing risks and multi-state models respectively. We address nonparametric estimation of the relevant quantities. In Chapters 4 and 5, we quantify the effect of covariables via regression models. In Chapter 4 we explain how and why the ideas and techniques of the classical Cox proportional hazards model extend to settings with competing risks and intermediate states. The difference is in the interpretation of the estimates and their translation to the cumulative scale. The latter is explained in Chapter 5. We also describe two approaches in which parameter estimates have a direct interpretation on the cumulative scale. One quantifies effects on another type of hazard, the subdistribution hazard. This model is often called the Fine and Gray model. The third uses a model that quantifies effects directly on the cumulative probability, the proportional odds model. Two of the main difficulties from a practical perspective are the translation of research questions into modeling choices and the interpretation of the results. Therefore, these issues are given a lot of attention throughout the book. The epilogue is completely devoted to this issue.

The last four sections of each chapter have the same structure. We first summarize the concepts that have been introduced, place them in a broader perspective and refer to issues that come up in subsequent chapters. The next section contains exercises that are intended to help understand and reflect on the concepts. Technical exercises are denoted by an asterisk. Answers to the exercises are provided at the end of the book. The exercises are followed by a section devoted to software. We briefly explain options in SAS and Stata. We give a detailed description of the functionality in the R statistical program [83]. Each chapter ends with computer practicals, in which you are asked to practice the concepts in R, using an existing data set on patients that underwent a bone marrow transplantation. In principle, all of the practicals on competing risks and some on multi-state models can also be made using Stata or SAS, but we do not provide any suggestions or answers.

Since we use examples from the biomedical and epidemiological field, the intended readership primarily consists of medical statisticians and epidemiologists. However, the book is useful for any researcher that has some experience with the analysis of standard time-to-event data and wants to extend knowledge and skills to the competing risks or multi-state setting. It should be easy to translate "individuals" and "diseases" to units and phenomena from one's own research area.

With respect to the topics covered and the intended readership, our book is most closely related to the book *Competing Risks and Multistate Models with R* [12]. That book takes a more theoretical perspective and relies fairly heavily on the description via counting processes, whereas our focus is more on interpretation. Yet, we also explain the techniques of estimation and inference and how they extend the setting of classical survival analysis with a single event type. We explain some of the more theoretical aspects in separate sections. Two important topics that are not covered in this book are the imputation of missing event types and estimation via the use of pseudo-values.

With respect to the use of R, we assume that one knows how to install a package, how to execute a script, how to select rows and columns, and we assume some familiarity with the use of functions and help files. In the example R code, we write down the full function name because this helps in finding the appropriate help file. For example, we write `summary.coxph`. Because of R's object orientation, it is sufficient to write `summary` when performing the analyses.

The book has a website, `http://www.competingrisks.org`, where you can find additional information. It has a file with hints for making the computer practicals (`ComputerExercisesRHints.pdf`) as well as a file with suggested R code, the resulting outcomes and explanatory text (`ComputerPracticalsAnswers.pdf`). It also contains a script file with all example code that is used in the book (`ExampleCode.R`) and gives information on upcoming courses.

Acknowledgements

The writing of this book has been a challenging and inspiring process, to which several persons have contributed. The book originates from the courses that I have been teaching together with Hein Putter. I borrowed several ideas on multi-state models from his slides and computer practicals. Johannes Mertsching provided some of the results in Chapter 2 while doing his internship. I thank the reviewers for their useful comments and suggestions, as well as my colleagues Marta Fiocco, Amy Matser and Jannie van der Helm for reading the first chapter of the book. Koos Zwinderman, you were right in saying that writing this book was going to be a weekend and evening job. Yet, I am grateful that you also gave me the opportunity to write parts of my book during office hours. I am convinced that it has been a profitable investment for the department as well. I also like to thank John Kimmel for allowing me to miss my deadline so many times, and Laurie Oknowsky and Michael Davidson for the editorial process.

I thank the Bikram yoga teachers for their tough classes, which filled me with new energy and creativity. Dear friends, you gave me mental support because you kept asking me about my progress. I hope I have been able to give you some idea of what the book is about. Yet, having finished the book does not mean that I will leave my laptop at home the next time. Jacquelien, I hope to open another bottle with white bubbles soon. Roberto, I have finally finished my "facebookie".

About the Author

Ronald Geskus received his Ph.D. in mathematical statistics at the Delft Technical University in 1997, based on a thesis entitled "Asymptotically efficient estimation with interval censored data" (supervisor Piet Groeneboom). Since 1995 he has been affiliated with the public health service of Amsterdam (PHS), where he performed and supervised studies on HIV and other sexually transmitted infections. There he specialized in the statistical analysis of data collected in cohort studies. In 2014 he was appointed associate professor at the Academic Medical Center (AMC) in Amsterdam. He has worked in several other medical and statistical research environments in the Netherlands and has spent sabbaticals in HIV/AIDS research groups in Paris and Madrid.

His research interests include: i) models for complex time-to-event data (competing risks, multi-state models), ii) models for complex longitudinal data, iii) prediction based on time-updated marker values, iv) causal inference. He contributed to and supervised many medical, epidemiological and statistical studies, performed both at the PHS and the AMC as well as within international collaborations.

He has published around 150 peer reviewed scientific articles, applied as well as methodological. He published methodological papers on i) the estimation of time from HIV infection to AIDS if the time of infection is unknown, ii) the development of markers in relation to disease progression, and iii) the analysis of competing risks with left truncated and right censored data. He is the joint first author of a highly cited tutorial on competing risks and multistate models.

He has been teaching courses on the analysis of competing risks data in Brazil, Spain, Belgium, Sweden, Austria and the Netherlands.

List of Figures

List of Tables

Symbol Description

$F(t)$	cumulative incidence function/net risk, all event types combined	$\widehat{F}^{\text{PL}}$	product-limit estimator of F (Kaplan-Meier)
$F_k(t)$	cause-specific cumulative incidence function/crude risk	$\widehat{F}^{\text{EC}}$	ECDF estimator of F
		$\widehat{F}_k^{\text{AJ}}$	Aalen-Johansen estimator of F_k
$\overline{F}$	$1 - F$, "survival" function. Similarly: $\overline{F_k} = 1 - F_k$ etc.	$\widehat{F}_k^{\text{PL}}$	product-limit estimator of F_k
$\text{P}_{gh}(s,t)$	transition probability	$\widehat{F}_k^{\text{EC}}$	ECDF estimator of F_k
T	random variable that has F as distribution: $T \sim F$	$\widehat{\Lambda}$	Nelson-Aalen estimator of cumulative hazard
T_k	random variable that has F_k as distribution: $T_k \sim F_k$	$t_{(i)}$	timing of i-th observed event (in numerical order)
C	time of censoring	$c_{(i)}$	timing of i-th observed censoring (in numerical order)
Γ	distribution of censoring time, $C \sim \Gamma$	$v_{(i)}$	timing of i-th observed entry (in numerical order)
L	entry time	$d(t)$	number of events, of any type, at time t
Φ	distribution of entry time, $L \sim \Phi$	$d_k(t)$	number of events of type k at time t
$h(t)$	overall hazard, all event types combined	$d_{gh}(t)$	number of transitions from g to h at time t
$h_k(t)$	subdistribution hazard	m_i	number of censorings at time $c_{(i)}$
$\lambda_k(t)$	cause-specific hazard		
$\lambda_{gh}(t)$	transition hazard	w_i	number of individuals entering the risk set at time $v_{(i)}$
$r(t)$	observed number at risk		
$r^*(t)$	number at risk in estimate of subdistribution hazard	$\widehat{N}$	virtual sample size, including missed individuals due to left truncation
$R(t)$	risk set		

Abbreviations

AIDS	acquired immune deficiency syndrome	ECDF	empirical cumulative distribution function
cART	combination anti-retroviral therapy	HCV	hepatitis C virus
		HIV	human immunodeficiency virus
CCR5	CC chemokine receptor 5		
CI	confidence interval	IDU	injecting drug user
COD	causes of death	MSM	men who have sex with men
EBMT	European group for bone and marrow transplantation	NSI	non syncytium inducing
		PL	product-limit
		SI	syncytium inducing

1

Basic Concepts

1.1 Introduction

Survival analysis techniques are used to answer questions about time to occurrence of events. An event is characterized by a transition from one state to another. In classical survival analysis there is only one initial state and only one event type, as shown schematically in Figure 1.1.

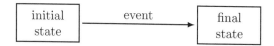

FIGURE 1.1
Schematic structure of the classical survival analysis setting.

Often, more can be learned by splitting events into types, which act as competing risks. For example, individuals with end stage renal disease that receive a kidney transplant have increased mortality shortly thereafter but reduced long-term mortality. The reason for this trend becomes clear once we distinguish causes of death: initial mortality is transplant related, but if a patient survives the first period he is less likely to die of renal failure than a patient that continues to be on dialysis.

Most events do not come unannounced. If we take intermediate events into account, we increase knowledge of the biological mechanisms leading to a final event and we can predict more accurately when the final event will happen. A multi-state model describes the sequence of events as transitions between states.

This chapter describes the basic concepts that play a role in survival analysis. Use of formulas is kept to a minimum. In Section 1.2, we describe the examples that are used in this book and formulate the questions of interest. The central role played by time brings about special characteristics of time-to-event data. The observation window during which data are collected typically causes individuals to have part of their disease history unobserved. In Section 1.3 we describe the most common forms of incomplete information: right censoring and left truncation. Survival analysis provides a toolbox to deal with such partially observed time-to-event data, a toolbox in which the hazard plays a predominant role. However, the hazard is not always the quantity of primary interest; often we want to quantify the probability that an event happens within a certain time span. In Section 1.4 we introduce the concepts of rate (hazard) and risk (cumulative probability) and extend them to the competing risks setting. (The extension to the multi-state setting is made in Section 3.2.) An important issue is whether the observation scheme is non-informative for the occurrence of the event. This is explained in more detail in Section 1.5. In Section 1.6 we relate the concepts of rate and risk and the necessary assumptions with respect to the observation scheme to the study questions from Section 1.2. Section 1.7 gives an overview of the notation that is used in this book. (Notation that is more specific for multi-state models is given in Section 3.2.1.) We summarize the most important notation in the Symbol Description list before this chapter. Section 1.8 gives a more formal overview of the main concepts and results from classical survival analysis.

1.2   Examples

The two main reasons to perform a statistical data analysis are to learn about etiology or causal effects and to improve prediction. Understanding etiology is a scientific activity that may have practical implications. Improving predictive performance is primarily useful for practice but is preferably based on a good etiologic model. Prediction can be at the individual level in clinical practice as well as at the population level. We give three examples. Later in this book we will see that the purpose of the study has impact on the choice of model and the assumptions that we have to make, and whether we consider only one event type or several types of events.

1.2.1   Infection during a hospital stay

During a hospital stay, some individuals become infected by the staphylococcus bacteria. Others are discharged from the hospital without having had an infection. The initial state is entered when an individual is admitted to hospital. From that state, individuals can progress to either infection or discharge as the first event. This is shown schematically in Figure 1.2. Individuals can also be discharged after staphylococcus infection or can get a staphylococcus infection outside the hospital, but these events are secondary and not of interest here.

Two different objectives are of interest. The etiologic objective is to quantify the infection risk. This reflects food hygienic conditions in the hospital. If all individuals would stay in the hospital forever, in the end everyone becomes infected: the cumulative probability of infection over time since admission starts at zero and increases to 100%. The other objective is to predict the

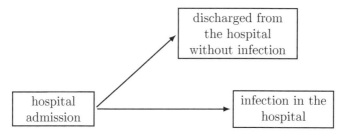

FIGURE 1.2
Example: staphylococcus infection during a hospital stay, with discharge without infection as competing event.

number of infections while staying in the hospital. This is important if we want to know the disease burden of infection during a hospital stay. Some individuals never become infected because they are discharged, and the cumulative probability of infection over time since admission will not reach 100%.

1.2.2 HIV infection

The human immunodeficiency virus (HIV) multiplies in CD4 T-cells. As a consequence, CD4 cell counts decrease. Because CD4 T-cells play an important role in our immune system, diseases develop that are not seen in healthy individuals. These diseases define the diagnosis Acquired Immune Deficiency Syndrome (AIDS). Without intervention, the median time from HIV infection to AIDS is around ten years. After the development of AIDS, most individuals die within a few years. The introduction of combination antiretroviral therapy (cART) in 1996 has dramatically changed the disease course.

We formulate three research questions, which we will try to answer using data from HIV/AIDS cohort studies.

1. Natural history. In the Western world, men who have sex with men (MSM) and injecting drug users (IDU) have been the most important risk groups for HIV infection. Because of their worse health status, IDUs may have a faster progression to AIDS. However, many IDUs don't develop AIDS because they die before. The situation is described in Figure 1.3.

We want to answer the etiologic question of whether the natural history of AIDS differs between MSM and IDUs. The natural history is the progression that would be observed if there were no interventions that change AIDS progression (like use of cART) or prevent AIDS from occurring (like pre-AIDS mortality).

2. Causes of death. The introduction of cART has caused a dramatic decrease in AIDS incidence and AIDS-related mortality. However, other causes of death are observed more frequently. Side effects of cART may increase mortality from causes such as cardiovascular disease. But even if cART itself

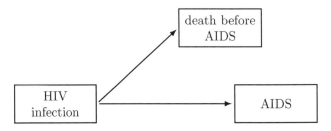

FIGURE 1.3
Example: progression from HIV infection to AIDS, with pre-AIDS mortality as competing event.

does not increase the risk of other causes of death, individuals that no longer die of AIDS will sooner or later die of something else. For example, the factors that increase the risk of HIV infection also increase the risk of hepatitis C virus (HCV) infection and anal infection by the human papilloma virus (HPV). HCV infection increases the risk of liver cancer, and some types of HPV can cause anal cancer. Both cancers can be lethal, but they often take much longer to develop than AIDS. As a consequence, they were rarely observed in the pre-cART era, when AIDS-related mortality was high.

The etiologic question is whether the biological effect of cART use is to increase other types of mortality. Another question is how the introduction of cART has changed the spectrum in observed causes of death, taking into account that other causes of death will occur more often if persons no longer die of AIDS. In Sections 4.6 and 5.3 we study both questions when we quantify the effects of HCV coinfection and the introduction of cART on different causes of death. The competing causes of death that we consider are depicted in Figure 1.4.

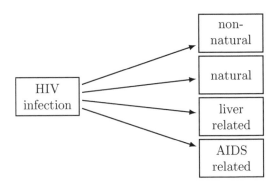

FIGURE 1.4
Example: spectrum in causes of death after HIV infection.

3. SI as intermediate event. During the course from HIV infection to death, intermediate events may occur that have an impact on subsequent disease progression. One such event is a switch of the HIV virus to the so-called syncytium inducing (SI) phenotype. In Figure 1.5 we describe the process from HIV infection to AIDS and death, with a switch to SI phenotype as a possible intermediate event.

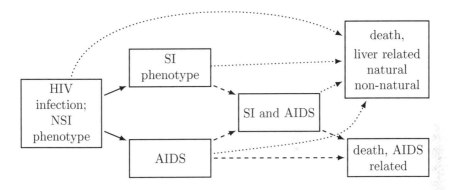

FIGURE 1.5
Example: progression from HIV infection to AIDS and death, with an SI switch as an intermediate event.

A deletion in the gene that codes for the C-C chemokine receptor 5 (CCR5) reduces susceptibility to HIV infection. This deletion is called CCR5-Δ32. Persons with the CCR5-Δ32 deletion on both chromosomes rarely become HIV infected. If the deletion is present on one of the chromosomes, HIV infection does occur but progression to AIDS is slower than for individuals in which both chromosomes do not have the deletion. The reason is that the HIV virus uses the CCR5 receptor for cell entry, and the deletion makes cell entry and multiplication more difficult. However, if the virus has switched to the SI phenotype, it can also use the CXC chemokine receptor 4 (CXCR4) for cell entry[1].

Little is known about factors that cause the SI phenotype to appear. Since in individuals with the CCR5-Δ32 deletion the non-SI (NSI) phenotype has more difficulties to replicate, it may be that the SI phenotype appears more rapidly. In Sections 4.3, 5.2.1 and 5.3.4 we will investigate this in a competing risks setting in which "AIDS before SI switch" acts as a competing event for "SI switch before AIDS" as the event of interest. The situation is depicted via the two solid arrows on the left-hand side of Figure 1.5. Just as in the example of causes of death, we will see that there are two approaches to answering this question; one is more etiologic, and the other is better suited for prediction.

Since neither of the events is final, we can also describe what happens

---

[1]Nowadays, CCR5-tropic and CXCR4-tropic virus are used as names instead of NSI and SI phenotype.

after the first event. This is depicted in Figure 1.5 by the states that are connected via dashed arrows (for HIV related events) and dotted arrows (for death due to other causes). The SI phenotype can also appear after AIDS diagnosis; therefore we need an arrow from AIDS to SI phenotype as well. The appearance of the SI phenotype worsens prognosis with respect to AIDS and death [38]. An interesting question is whether the protective effect of the CCR5-Δ32 deletion on progression to AIDS and death is still present after the virus has switched to the SI phenotype. In Sections 4.5 and 5.2.2 we use a multi-state model to quantify how the risk of AIDS changes after the switch to SI phenotype and whether progression to AIDS and death after the SI switch differs by CCR5 genotype. We will also investigate the effect of age on the occurrence of the different events.

Note that Figures 1.3 and 1.4 can be seen as special cases of Figure 1.5. Depending on the question of interest, some states are left out and some are combined. In Figure 1.3, the states "SI phenotype" and "death, AIDS related" are left out; all three causes of death that are not AIDS related are taken together and the states "AIDS" and "SI and AIDS" are combined into one state "AIDS". In Figure 1.4, SI switch and AIDS are not considered as intermediate events.

1.2.3 Bone marrow transplantation

Bone marrow transplantation is one of the ways to treat patients with leukemia. The process after allogeneic bone marrow transplantation, i.e. transplantation from a genetically non-identical donor, can be described via the states as in Figure 1.6. An adverse event is the acute reaction of the immune

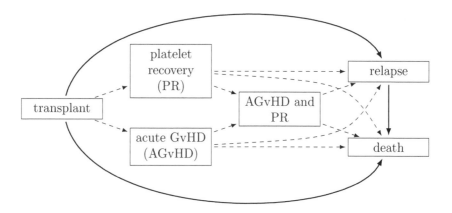

FIGURE 1.6
Example: events after bone marrow transplantation.

system in the donor graft against normal host tissues, which is called acute graft-versus-host disease (AGvHD). Another intermediate event is relapse, and death is the final event. A beneficial event is the recovery of platelet counts to normal levels.

All these states have been used to model and predict the disease course after transplantation [28]. A simplified version was used in a tutorial on competing risks [81]: AGvHD was ignored and relapse and death were combined into one state.

In the computer practicals we only consider relapse as a possible intermediate state on the pathway to death. Hence we leave out the states in the middle and can describe our model via the states that are connected via the solid arrows in Figure 1.6. We investigate the role of the EBMT risk score[2]. This score is a combination of donor-recipient match and age of the recipient, among other things. It divides patients into three risk groups. We quantify the effect of the EBMT score on all three transitions and we test whether the effects on the transitions are different. We also investigate whether progression from relapse to death depends on year of relapse. Treatment of relapse has improved over time, and some clinicians have gone so far as to suggest that having a relapse does not influence mortality anymore.

1.3   Data structure

The principal information per individual consists of a series of states in which he has been and the times at which he has entered and left these states. Time is always quantified with respect to some reference value, the time origin, that determines the time scale (Section 1.3.1). Typically, in some individuals only part of the relevant time scale is observed. If the final part of the time scale is not observed, an event time is right censored (Section 1.3.2). Left truncation is a phenomenon that may arise if the individual is not observed in the beginning of the time scale (Section 1.3.3).

1.3.1   Time scales

Data is collected in calendar time. Calendar time is also the time scale of interest for the analysis if we want to investigate the development of an epidemic like HIV. The standard reference value of calendar time in a large part of the world is the start of the Christian calendar. Statistical packages by default choose another origin when representing calendar time[3].

More often, the time scale of interest is initiated by the occurrence of some

---

[2]EBMT stands for European Group for Bone and Marrow Transplantation.

[3]SPSS uses October 14, 1582 (the start of the Gregorian calendar), Stata uses January 1st, 1960 and R uses January 1st, 1970.

event in the person. Examples of such events are birth, hospital admission, HIV infection, AIDS diagnosis, the start of cART and bone marrow transplantation. Study entry can also initialize a time scale, but this scale usually has little biological or epidemiological interest.

Figure 1.7 gives a schematic description of these two time scales. In the upper part, an individual is shown that entered the study on March 6th 1995. The event that initiates the process of interest happened more than three years later, on July 8th 1998. Another four years later, on November 11th 2002, the event occurred that defines the end point. In the lower part, we show his personal time scale. In this time scale, the initiating event defines the time origin. Note that the calendar time at which the initiating event occurs generally differs per person. If the study entry had been after the initiating event, a correction for left truncation may be needed (Section 1.3.3), but again, study entry itself does not generate a time scale of interest.

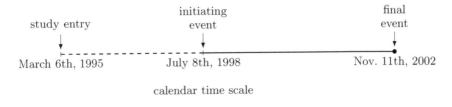

calendar time scale

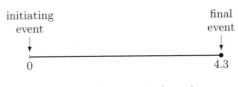

personal time scale (years)

FIGURE 1.7
Events in the calendar time scale and the personal time scale.

Concerning the choice of time scale, competing risks analysis is not different from classical survival analysis; the difference between both is not in the event that initiates the time scale, but in the number of event types that can serve as an end point. In the multi-state setting, multiple time scales may play a role. The occurrence of an intermediate event may generate another relevant time scale: time since entering that state.

1.3.2 Right censored data

An individual is right censored with respect to an event if he were observed to be at risk for experiencing the event during some time but the event itself was not observed. We distinguish between three types of right censored data.

Administrative censoring This occurs if individuals are still in follow-up without having experienced the event yet. Usually the administrative censoring time is based on a fixed calendar date that is chosen as the end of follow-up for the analysis, aptly named "date of analysis". All information after this date is not taken into consideration. On a personal time scale the administrative censoring time will differ per individual, unless all individuals had the initiating event at the same calendar date. In the statistical literature administrative censoring has been called progressive type I censoring [6].

Loss to follow-up Individuals are lost to follow-up if they stopped being under observation before the date of analysis and before the event occurred. This can happen for several reasons. They may have moved to another country, they may have lost motivation to continue in the study or they may have become too ill to continue participation.

Competing risk A competing risk is another event that prevents the event of interest from happening. The most straightforward example is when an individual dies and death is not in the definition of the event of interest, such as with pre-AIDS mortality in HIV infected individuals. It may also be that an individual can still experience the event, but another event has happened first that changes the conditions under which the event of interest can occur. This has been called artificial censoring [48]. Examples of artificial censoring are discharge from hospital if infection during the hospital stay is the event of interest, AIDS before SI switch if SI switch before AIDS is the event of interest, or the start of cART if the natural history to AIDS is the event of interest.

Each of the three types differs with respect to the occurrence and possible observation of the event. With administrative censoring, the event may be observed in the future if the study is still ongoing. With loss to follow-up, the event may have occurred already before the date of analysis, but if so it was not observed. With competing risks, the event of interest will never happen.

This classification of types of censored data is relevant for several reasons. First, it may help in determining whether censoring is informative for progression to the event of interest (see Section 1.5). Second, censoring due to the occurrence of a competing event is interpreted differently from the other types of censoring in a competing risks analysis (see e.g. Section 1.4 and Chapter 6). Third, administrative censoring can be treated in a special way in some estimation methods for competing risks data (see Section 2.4.3.2). This is because the administrative censoring time is always known, also if the individual experienced a competing event before. In a competing risks setting, data in which all other censoring is administrative, i.e. data in which there is no loss to follow-up, has been called censoring complete data [34].

If an event occurs, its exact timing may be known even if the individual has not been followed continuously. This is usually the case with directly observable event types such as admission to or discharge from the hospital, transplantation, and mortality. Even if the person is only seen intermittently, information on the timing of such an event can be recovered retrospectively. For other event types, information on the event status is only known at the observation times. We may know that the event happened in-between two observation times, but the exact timing is unknown. This is called interval censored data. Examples of such event types are HIV infection and switch to SI phenotype. The analysis of interval censored data is more complex and the methodology is not well-developed yet. If the interval is narrow compared to the total time range within which events can occur, an alternative approach is to make an approximation. For example, one can take the midpoint of the interval and treat this as an exactly observed event time. For HIV infection, the midpoint between the last HIV negative test and first HIV positive test is often assumed as date of infection[4]. This is a reasonable approximation if the end point takes years to happen, as is the case with the development of AIDS after HIV infection.

Data is left censored if the the event happened before the first observation time. If all events are either left censored or observed exactly, analysis can be performed by reversing the time scale. Left censored data is much less common than right censored data.

1.3.3   Left truncated data

A typical example of left truncated data is found in cohort studies with late entry: some individuals enter the study after the event that defines the origin of the personal time scale. As an example, consider the data from the Amsterdam Cohort Studies on HIV Infection and AIDS (ACS). These studies were started in October 1984, shortly after the first test to detect HIV infection had become available. Suppose that an individual became infected in September 1981[5]. If he entered the ACS in January 1985 and died as a consequence of HIV infection in May 1989, his time and event information is as illustrated in Figure 1.8. In his personal time scale, he entered the study 3.34 years after HIV infection.

Left truncation is present when the data is subject to a form of length biased sampling: individuals that became HIV infected at the beginning of the epidemic and had a short time to AIDS and death are missed. The information with respect to both the calendar time of HIV infection and the personal time from HIV infection to death can be shown graphically as in Figure 1.9. A fast progressor that became infected in 1980 and died before the study started, for example in July 1984, did not have the possibility to enter the study. The grey area represents the "unobserved" period: all the combinations of the

---

[4]Since HIV infection is usually determined via the presence of HIV specific antibodies, HIV seroconversion is the real time origin. However, time between HIV infection and HIV seroconversion is almost always less than three months, which is short compared to the average time from HIV infection to AIDS and death. We will continue to speak of time since infection instead of seroconversion.

[5]This may be known through information from stored blood samples.

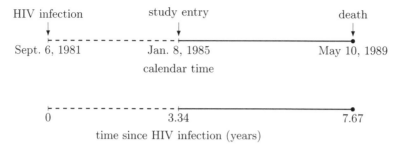

FIGURE 1.8
Late entry in calendar time scale and personal time scale.

infection date and the subsequent time to death that make it impossible to enter the study because death occurred before the study started. Not only HIV infected individuals that died before the start of the study will be missed. The same holds for any HIV infected individual that died before he would enter the study. For example, the individual from Figure 1.8 entered the study on January 8, 1985 and would have been missed as well if he had died between the start of the ACS at the end of October 1984 and his time of entry. The

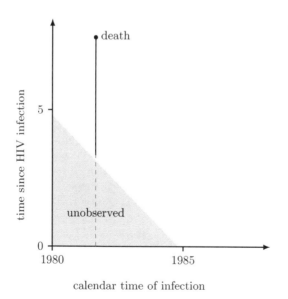

FIGURE 1.9
Graphical representation of left truncation via the event space. Grey triangle: unobserved period. Vertical line: individual from Figure 1.8; the dashed line becomes a solid line from his moment of entry onwards.

shorter the time from HIV infection to death, the more likely it is that an individual is missed. This is the mechanism behind length-biased sampling.

Left truncation also occurs in studies in which age, i.e. time since birth, is the principal time scale. Individuals often have not been followed from birth onwards and may be missed if they experienced the event of interest before they could enter the study.

In general, there is left truncation with respect to an event if both of the following conditions hold i) there are individuals that came under observation for the event some time after they became at risk for experiencing the event and ii) they would be missed if the event had happened before they came under observation for the event.

There are situations in which the first condition holds, but the second does not. Suppose time from HIV infection until AIDS is studied on an island with only one hospital. Individuals enter the study when they visit the hospital and turn out to be HIV infected. Although there is late entry, the event would never be missed if all HIV infected individuals end up in hospital.

Another mechanism that generates a form of left truncated data is when some characteristic of an individual that changes over time is included in the analysis. Examples are the inclusion of a time-varying covariable in a regression model (see Section 1.8.5) or an intermediate state in a multi-state model (see Chapter 3). In fact, as explained in Section 4.5.2, entering a state can be seen and analysed as a change in time-varying covariable. One of the simplest examples of a time-varying covariable is calendar time of follow-up (see Figure 1.17 on Page 41). An individual that experiences the initiating event in an earlier calendar period becomes at risk for experiencing the end point of interest in the later calendar period only some time after his time origin. If he had experienced the event in the earlier calendar period, he would not be included in the risk set—he would be missed—for the later period. This type of truncation has been called internal left truncation [6].

Often, left truncation and left censoring are mixed up. Truncation and censoring are different mechanisms. With censoring, part of the observation period is missing, but every individual is as likely to be included in the sample. With truncation, some individuals are missed completely. In HIV/AIDS cohort studies, an individual may enter the study some time after HIV infection. If the exact time of infection is unknown, entry time into the "infection" state is left censored. If HIV infection itself is the event of interest, it is a left censored end point. If time from HIV infection to AIDS is the quantity of interest, it is a left censored time origin. If the time origin is left censored, then there is late entry with respect to the time from HIV infection to AIDS and a left truncation mechanism is likely to be present as well[6]. If the date of HIV infection is known for every individual in the analysis, also for the ones who entered after HIV infection, then there is left truncation but no left censoring.

---

[6]Left truncation is absent in the example above of the island with one hospital.

Note that an individual can have both a late entry time and a right censored final event time.

Another mechanism is right truncation. Right truncated data does not occur very often, but in Section 2.4.2 we encounter a situation. If there is only right truncated data, no left truncated data, estimation can be performed by reversing the time scale.

We restrict to methods for right censored and left truncated data, and refer to the literature for estimation using more complicated observation schemes.

1.4   On rates and risks

The time component allows for two different quantifications: instantaneous and cumulative.

The instantaneous measure is the fraction of individuals that develops an event at some time, amongst the ones that are at risk for experiencing the event at that time. In epidemiology, it is commonly called the rate, but when the event is a disease, the term incidence is used as well. It is also been called the risk, but we reserve that word for the cumulative measure. The statistical name is the hazard, which is the one that we will use most in this book.

The cumulative measure is the fraction of individuals that develops an event within some time span, amongst the ones that are at risk for experiencing the event at the start of that time period. For a meaningful interpretation it requires the start of the time period to be synchronized for every individual. Therefore, for many processes it cannot be used in the calendar time scale; the cumulative fraction of persons with diabetes cannot be defined if new persons enter the risk set during calendar time. Because it is a cumulative probability, the cumulative incidence never decreases if the time span increases. In epidemiology it is commonly called cumulative incidence or (actuarial) risk. The statistical name is the cumulative distribution function. It is the complement of the survival function, i.e. one minus the survival function. In this book, we use the names cumulative incidence and risk.

Due to the presence of right censored and left truncated data, the analysis of time-to-event data is easier via the hazard. As a consequence, most models and estimation methods are based on the hazard. Examples are the Kaplan-Meier estimate of the survival function and the Cox proportional hazards regression model (see Section 1.8). In classical survival analysis with one type of end point, hazard and cumulative incidence are related via a one-to-one relation: if we know one, we also know the other. An important consequence of this relation is that the effect of a covariable as quantified via a regression model for the hazard translates to a similar effect on the cumulative incidence.

Both measures can be extended to the settings with competing risks and intermediate states. These are characterized by the presence of several event types, which can be analysed and interpreted in different ways. In the presence of competing risks, we distinguish between a marginal analysis, a competing risks analysis, and a combined analysis.

In a marginal analysis we are interested in one specific event type. We want to quantify the hazard and cumulative incidence that would be observed if the competing events did not occur. For example, we quantify the rate and risk of staphylococcus infection that would be observed if everyone would stay in hospital. We use the names marginal hazard for the rate and marginal cumulative incidence or net risk for the cumulative measure.

In a competing risks analysis we want to quantify the progression to a specific event type, taking into account that individuals can also progress to other end points. The cumulative progression over time to the event of interest has been given many different names: absolute risk, crude risk, cause-specific cumulative incidence (function), crude cumulative incidence (function), crude incidence curve, crude probability function, actual probability, cause-specific risk, cause-specific failure probability, subdistribution function and even just cumulative incidence. We will use the names cause-specific cumulative incidence, crude risk and subdistribution function. It is called a subdistribution function because it is not a proper distribution: as time progresses its value does not increase from zero to one because a competing event can prevent the event of interest from happening.

In a competing risks analysis, two hazards can be defined. There is a hazard that has the one-to-one relation with the cause-specific cumulative incidence. It is most often called the subdistribution hazard or subhazard. It has the somewhat awkward definition as the fraction of individuals that develops the event of interest at some time point, amongst the individuals that either are at risk or have already experienced a competing event (see definition (2.8) and the discussion in Section 2.7). A second hazard type is closer to the standard rate concept: it is the fraction of individuals that develops the event of interest at some time point amongst those that are still at risk of experiencing the event (see definition (2.1)). It is most often called the cause-specific hazard, although other names have been used as well (even subhazard). It does not have a one-to-one relation with the cause-specific cumulative incidence (see Section 2.2.1). As a consequence, the way in which covariables are associated with a cause-specific hazard may not coincide with the way in which these covariables are associated with the cause-specific cumulative incidence (see Section 5.2.1 for an example). Note that, if only one event type is of interest, all competing event types can be collapsed into one "other" event type.

We can also combine all event types into one. For example, instead of discriminating between causes of death, we look at overall mortality. Then we are back in the classical setting of a single event type without competing risks. We will use the names overall hazard and overall cumulative incidence for this quantity. The overall hazard is equal to the sum of the cause-specific hazards and the overall cumulative incidence is equal to the sum of the cause-specific cumulative incidences (see Section 2.2.1). If death and some other event are competing end points, the cumulative probability to remain free of both end points is often called the event-free survival. The combined end point plays a role in estimation of the cause-specific cumulative incidence.

The four types of hazards and the corresponding cumulative quantities are summarized in Table 1.1.

TABLE 1.1

Hazard types and corresponding cumulative measures in the presence of multiple end points

	hazard		cumulative	
competing risks	marginal	*	net risk marginal cumulative incidence marginal survival function	*
	cause-specific	λ_k	no corresponding quantity	
	subdistribution	h_k	crude risk subdistribution function cause-specific cumulative incidence	$F_k(t)$
combined	overall	h	overall risk overall cumulative incidence overall survival function	$F(t)$

* Doesn't play a role in competing risks analyses; therefore, no notation is introduced

In a multi-state setting, only the transition hazard is used as instantaneous quantity. It is defined as the fraction of individuals that progresses from state A to state B at some time point, amongst the ones that are in state A. It has the same interpretation as the cause-specific hazard. Several cumulative measures can be defined. The basic one is called the transition probability. It is defined for any combination of states between which transitions, direct or indirect, can occur and for any two time points. It quantifies the fraction of individuals that is in state B at some time, amongst the ones that were in state A at some earlier time point. All transition hazards together describe the multi-state process, but again there is no one-to-one relation with the transition probability. Formal definitions of these and some other measures are given in Section 3.2.1.

1.5   Non-informative observation schemes?

We turn to estimation of the measures that were described in Section 1.4. Unbiased estimation requires some assumptions with respect to the right censoring and left truncation mechanisms. When right censoring is caused by a competing risk, the assumptions differ between a marginal analysis and a competing risks analysis. For left truncation due to late entry, the necessary assumptions are the same for both types of analyses. The assumptions that are required in a multi-state model are given in Section 3.3.2.

Right censored data

We first concentrate on the assumptions with respect to right censoring in a setting without competing risks. Since there is only one event type, there is only one type of hazard[7]. When estimating the hazard, an individual is removed from the risk set at the time he is right censored for the event. We assume that he can be represented by the individuals that remain in follow-up, in the sense that the distribution of his residual event time is the same. This assumption is valid if the fact that an individual leaves the study without the event of interest having happened does not provide any information with respect to his future event time: censoring is non-informative.

If there are no competing risks, all censoring is administrative or due to loss to follow-up. Every censored individual has an event time, which is larger than his censoring time. One way to model non-informative censoring is by assuming that every individual that has the event observed also has a censoring time. In this way, we can define a bivariate distribution for the event and censoring times. Non-informative censoring now means that the time-to-censoring distribution and the time-to-event distribution are independent[8].

We can visualize independent censoring via a scatter plot. Suppose that we follow individuals for a maximum of ten months. Death is the event of interest. After three months it is decided that the study will continue with half of the participants that are still alive. They are selected at random. Hence, censoring is non-informative. In the left panel of Figure 1.10, the event times and censoring times are shown for the individuals that were still alive after three months. The diagonal line is the line for which x and y have the same value. The event and censoring times of the individuals that leave the study after three months are shown by the grey points along the horizontal line at $y = 3$. Since censoring is non-informative, their (unobserved) death times have approximately the same distribution as the (observed) death times of individuals that continue to be in follow-up until year ten (the black points). Hence, in order to quantify mortality after three months, the censored individuals can be represented by the individuals that remain under observation.

Since the decision on censoring is not made for individuals that died within three months, strictly speaking they did not have a censoring time. But an equivalent situation would arise if the decision on censoring at three months were made at random at the start of the study. Then also the individuals that died in the first three months would have a censoring time. The right panel of Figure 1.10 shows how the complete data on censoring and event time for

---

[7]We could call it a marginal hazard.

[8]Sometimes, non-informative censoring and independent censoring are defined in slightly different ways [6, Definition III.2.2].

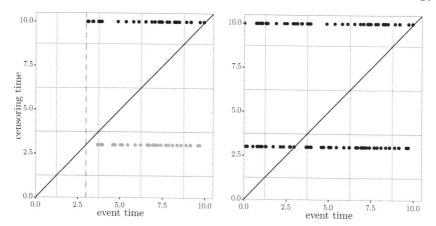

FIGURE 1.10

Graphical representation of non-informative censoring. Left panel: information beyond three months; individuals leaving the study at three months are in gray. Right panel: complete data until ten months.

the first ten months could have been. Independence between censoring time and event time is reflected by the absence of a correlation in the scatterplot of the complete data.

If we want to perform a marginal analysis in the presence of competing risks, the same independence assumption should hold for censoring due to the competing risks. We want to quantify the distribution for the situation without the competing risks. For unbiased estimation, we need to assume that those that are censored due to a competing risk can be represented by the ones that remain in follow-up.

However, if we perform a competing risks analysis, censoring due to competing risks is not required to be non-informative. The reason is that censoring due to the occurrence of a competing event has a different interpretation: such censored individuals are not supposed to be represented by the ones that remain in follow-up. We do not want to quantify progression to the event of interest if the competing events would not exist. We quantify the rates and risks of the event, taking into account that individuals can also experience some other event instead.

We may try to use the data to test for non-informative censoring. Unfortunately, it has been shown that this is not possible [103]. The reason is that, if an individual is right censored, we do not know whether the event would have happened the day after or many years later. We give a graphical argument by showing that the same observed data with respect to event time and censoring time can be generated by a mechanism in which they are independent as well as by one in which they are dependent. Hence, the observed data does not allow us to discriminate between both.

Again, we first consider the situation without competing risks, such that every individual can be assumed to have both an event time and a censoring time. The combination of event time and censoring time follows some bivariate distribution, just like weight and height do. Data on weight and height from a sample of individuals could be as in the scatterplot A of Figure 1.11. In subfigure B, exactly the same points as in subfigure A are plotted, but now they refer to event times and censoring times. The difference in the survival setting is that we only observe one, the earliest, of the event times and censoring times. For the other time, we only know that it occurs later. Because the data is only partially observed, it is plotted in grey. For example, the arrow in subfigure B points to an event time that is not observed because censoring occurred first. We do know the censoring time, which is read from the y-axis. For the event time we only know that it has some value along the horizontal dashed line that starts at the diagonal and crosses the unobserved true event time. Hence for every individual, the observed information consists of either a horizontal line (right censored event) or a vertical line (event observed, censoring time is larger). The information that we observe is shown in subfigure C. In subfigure D, we add points again in such a way that they are still in correspondence with the observed information in subfigure C. For example, the point with the arrow has moved to the right along the horizontal line. In subfigure E, we remove the lines and the scatterplot is seen to correspond to a situation in which event time and censoring time are independent.

In summary, if individuals experienced the event shortly after they were censored (as in A/B), such that censoring time and event time were dependent, this would lead to the same observed data (as in C) as in a situation of independence between the time-to-event and time-to-censoring distributions (which could generate a pattern as in D/E). Hence, the observed data does not allow us to decide which of the two (or any other degree of dependence) is the real one. If censoring is due to a competing risk, the event of interest will never occur but the same property holds.

Left truncated data

With left truncation due to late entry we need to make a similar assumption in order to obtain unbiased estimates. At every time point, individuals that are in follow-up and event-free should have the same future event risk as individuals that have not entered the study (yet) at that time point. And the fact that an individual enters the study event-free should not provide any information with respect to his future event time. Then, the unobserved individuals can be represented by the ones that are in follow-up.

Similar to right censoring, one way to model non-informative left truncation is by defining a distribution for the entry times that is independent from the time-to-entry distribution. This refers to the distribution of the whole sample, including the individuals that are not observed because they experienced the event before entry.

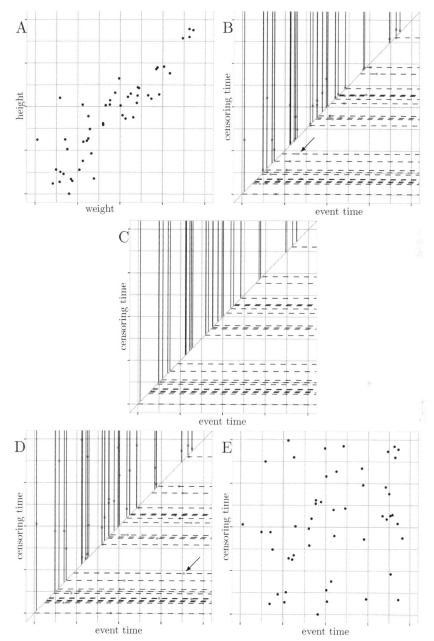

FIGURE 1.11

Graphical explanation why we cannot decide from the observed data whether the censoring time and event time distributions are independent.

Although it has been claimed otherwise [52], we cannot establish whether event time and entry time are independent based on the observed data. We show this in Figure 1.12 for a situation without right censored data; in the presence of right censored data the argument is not different, but slightly harder to visualize. We assume a bivariate distribution for the event times and entry times. In (A) entry times and event times are dependent, whereas in (B) they are independent. The only individuals that are included in the sample are the ones for whom the event time is larger than the entry time. These are the points in the lower right triangle of Figure 1.12. The grey points in the upper triangle are not observed. Based on the observed data, we cannot tell whether (A) or (B) holds.

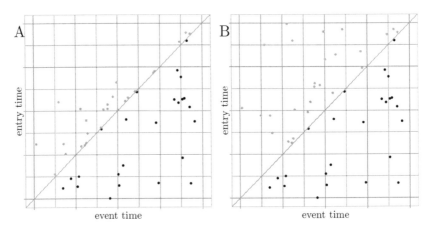

FIGURE 1.12
Graphical explanation why we cannot decide from the observed data whether the event time and entry time distributions are independent.

A difference with right censored data is that the observed information in the lower right triangle consists of points instead of lines. We can test for some form of independence in the lower triangle [102]. However, we need the entry times and the event times also to be independent over the unobserved region.

1.5.1 Some possible solutions

We cannot determine whether right censoring or left truncation is non-informative based on the data of the event times and entry or censoring times. So what can we do?

We may observe right censoring or late entry to be informative. For right censoring, this can only be established by using extra information. If we have a variable that is associated with both the event time and the censoring time, it induces dependence between both. Informative late entry may already be observed via the data on entry time and event time as in Figure 1.12. If we observe a clear correlation between the points in the lower triangle, then the relation in the upper triangle is no longer relevant and we can conclude that entry time and event time are dependent.

If we observe that one or more variables induce dependence, we can include them in our analyses. One approach is to include them as covariables in a regression model. Then we quantify the event time distribution conditionally on the value of the covariables. Due to non-collapsibility of the hazard [41], the estimates thus obtained are different from the population values. If we want to estimate the values for the population, we can use inverse probability weights instead [85, 89, 70, 48]. In this approach, we first construct a model for the probability to enter or to be censored based on the covariables that are responsible for the dependence. Based on this model, individuals that are observed to be at risk are reweighted by the estimated probability to have entered and not to be censored (yet).

But we can never be sure that such a correction is sufficient to make the observation scheme non-informative, which is what we need. There may be other variables that cause the observation scheme still to be informative. A non-informative observation scheme will remain an assumption that cannot be verified based on data. This is similar to the situation in causal inference and with missing data. We never know whether we corrected for all the relevant confounders or whether we included all important covariables in the imputation procedure.

If we don't have information on variables that explain the dependence, another approach is to specify some relation between entry/censoring time and event time, e.g. by means of copulas. This has been compared with an approach based on censoring weights [107]. Again, correctness of the relation cannot be verified based on the data.

The use of copulas has been advocated in semi-competing risk settings [32]. Semi-competing risks occur if the event of interest does not terminate follow-up. As a consequence, the competing event can also be observed after the occurrence of the event of interest. An example is the estimation of time from start of cART until virological failure in HIV infected individuals, with dropout as the competing event. The situation is shown schematically in Figure 1.13: follow-up ends at dropout, but dropout may also occur after virological failure.

In Figure 1.14, the observable event time information is shown graphically for two situations[9]. If virological failure occurs first, we can observe both event times (the upper triangle). If dropout occurs first, we only know that virological failure may occur later (lower triangle). Based on this information, the marginal distribution of the competing event, dropout, can be estimated. And the relation between both event types is observed in the upper triangle. If we are willing to assume that the observed relation can be extended to

---

[9]We use the same scatterplot as in Figures 1.11 and 1.12 and assume that there is no left truncation nor other types of censoring.

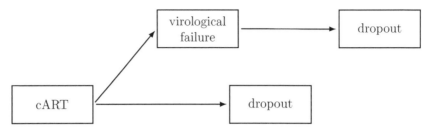

FIGURE 1.13
Typical situation of semi-competing risks: the event of interest, virological failure, does not terminate follow-up.

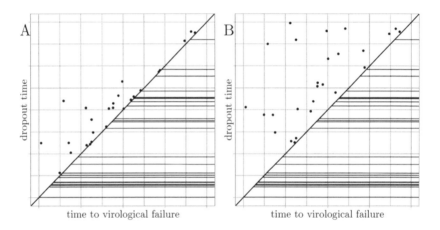

FIGURE 1.14
Graphical representation of semi-competing risks data.

the lower triangle, we can estimation the bivariate distribution as well as the marginal distribution of the event of interest.

Note that the example in Figure 1.13 can also be analysed as an illness-death multi-state model (see Section 3.2). Then we do not quantify the marginal distribution of virological failure but the transition hazards and transition probabilities among the three different states.

A third option is to argue why we think a non-informative observation scheme is a reasonable assumption. For right censored data, it helps to have another look at the three general reasons for censoring.

Administrative censoring Often, the assumption that censoring is independent is a reasonable one. An individual that entered the study four months before the date of analysis is censored after four months if still event-free. His unobserved residual time-to-event distribution is likely to be the same as that from an individual that entered the study at a much earlier date, was event-free four months later, and remained in follow-up. The assumption does not hold when there is some calendar time trend in the event time distribution. In that situation, an individual that entered shortly before the date of analysis has a different event time distribution than an individual that entered much earlier. Correcting for calendar period solves this problem.

Loss to follow-up Censoring may be informative. If individuals leave the study because they become too ill to continue follow-up, they are closer to the event than the individuals that do not leave the study. Or if individuals that are healthy feel less need to continue participation or move to another country, they are less likely to develop the event than the individuals that remain in the study.

Competing risk Usually there is some biological mechanism that influences progression to the different event types and we cannot assume that censoring is independent. As mentioned before, this type of censoring is allowed to be informative if we perform a competing risks analysis.

The entry time is informative if individuals enter the study for reasons that are related to disease progression. We give two examples. Suppose we are interested in the time from HIV infection to AIDS and use data from a hospital-based cohort study. Individuals enter the study when they visit the hospital and they turn out to be HIV positive. Individuals may have visited the hospital because they experienced the consequences of their HIV infection. For example, it may be that the individual in Figure 1.8 visited the hospital because he had had a fever for several weeks. His subsequent AIDS risk will be higher than the average AIDS risk for individuals that are AIDS-free after 3.34 years. Note that informative late entry may not lead to informative left truncation if it is the only hospital on an island (see Page 12). Another example of informative late entry is the estimation of age at death based on data from individuals that entered a retirement center (see e.g. the Channing data set in Klein & Moeschberger [55]). The fact that they entered a retirement center is related to progression to death. Informative late entry is also the reason for the bias when using one of the entry criteria in Exercise 8 on Page 49.

1.6 The examples revisited

1.6.1 Infection during a hospital stay

In the staphylococcus example, we formulated two different research aims. One was etiologic: to quantify the impact of the hygienic conditions in the hospital on staphylococcus infection. The other was to predict how many infections are to be expected in the hospital.

When answering the etiologic question, we estimate the marginal distribution. We estimate the cumulative percentage of infections over time—the net risk or (marginal) cumulative incidence—that is observed if discharge did not occur and everyone remained in hospital. The time scale of the process is short. If we define discharge in a broad sense and include mortality during hospital stay, everyone has either of the competing events observed. For infection as the event, the only censoring is due to the competing risk discharge. The net risk is estimated via the Kaplan-Meier procedure. It is based on the estimator of the marginal hazard, in which individuals are removed from the risk set upon discharge (see Section 1.8.2). It is a valid estimator of the marginal hazard only if individuals that are discharged can be represented by the individuals that remain in follow-up. If the discharged individuals had remained in hospital, they should have had the same infection risk as the ones that actually did remain in hospital: censoring due to discharge is non-informative. Non-informative censoring is a reasonable assumption if the infection rate is the same for every individual. If this is not the case, the Kaplan-Meier curve does not represent an interpretable quantity and the marginal distribution cannot be estimated without incorporating extra information or making additional assumptions.

For prediction of what actually happens, we interpret discharge as a competing risk. We estimate the cumulative probability of infection in the hospital—the crude risk or cause-specific cumulative incidence—in the actual situation that individuals can also experience another type of event instead, discharge without infection. Once an individual is discharged without infection, he can no longer become infected in the hospital. We don't assume that individuals that are discharged can be represented by the ones that remain in the hospital.

When comparing two hospitals, results of the marginal analysis may differ from results of the competing risks analysis. If the infection rate is the same in both hospitals but the rate of discharge is different, the marginal distribution of infection is the same, but fewer infections will be observed in the hospital in which the rate of discharge is larger. In the latter hospital, more individuals leave the hospital before they would be infected. A similar example in which effects are different is given in Section 5.2.

1.6.2   HIV infection

1. Natural history. In the first HIV example, we want to answer the etiologic question of whether the distribution of time from HIV infection to AIDS differs between MSM and IDUs. This is quantified by the marginal distribution of time to AIDS. We use the Kaplan-Meier procedure and make individuals leave the risk set when they die before AIDS diagnosis. The result is shown in Figure 1.15.

The curves suggest that injecting drugs slows down progression to AIDS. This is unlikely to be true. The shallower curve for the IDUs is probably not due to some biological mechanism, but due to informative censoring. In

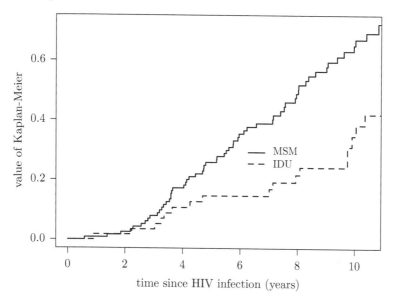

FIGURE 1.15
Kaplan-Meier curves for progression to AIDS on the complementary scale "one-minus-survival".

the computation of the Kaplan-Meier curve, individuals that died before AIDS leave the risk set. In order to interpret the result as an estimate of the marginal distribution, we assume that they can be represented by the IDUs that did not die. The data on time to AIDS and death does not allow us to see whether censoring due to death is informative or not. However, additional information was available on the causes of death. In Table 1.2 we see that 17 out of the 99 IDUs died and some of the causes of death were related to AIDS progres-

TABLE 1.2
Observed causes of death before AIDS diagnosis

| | IDU | MSM |
Cause of death	Number	
HIV related infections	3	0
overdose/suicide	6	0
violence/accident	2	0
liver cirrhosis	2	0
cancer	0	1
heart attack	0	1
unknown	4	3

sion. They were not far from developing AIDS and therefore they cannot be represented by the IDUs that did not die: pre-AIDS death is informative for AIDS. Therefore, the Kaplan-Meier curve for the IDUs does not reflect the marginal distribution of time from HIV infection to AIDS. In fact, it has no interpretation. Among the MSM, only 5 out of 127 died, and the causes of death were less clearly related to AIDS progression.

An alternative approach that circumvents the problem of informative censoring due to pre-AIDS mortality is to analyse pre-AIDS death as a competing risk. In Figure 1.16, we plot the estimates of the cumulative fraction of individuals that progress to AIDS and that die before developing AIDS, the crude risks or cause-specific cumulative incidences. This estimator is explained in Chapter 2.

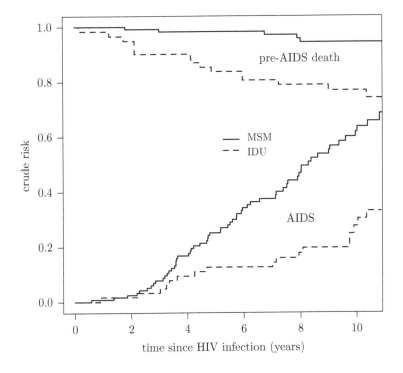

FIGURE 1.16
Estimates of cause-specific cumulative incidence for AIDS and pre-AIDS death.

In order to increase visibility, the estimate for pre-AIDS mortality is plotted on the survival scale, going down from the value one (this is called the alternate display format, see Page 66). We see that within 8 years about 50% of the MSM developed AIDS whereas this percentage was only 20% for IDUs.

On the other hand, within 8 years 20% of the IDUs died before AIDS diagnosis and less than 5% of the MSM died.

These curves answer a different question; they predict the cumulative AIDS risk in a situation in which individuals can also experience death as a competing event. Since many deaths were the consequence of an intervention, the curves do not quantify the biological mechanism of progression to AIDS and therefore cannot be used if we want to compare the natural history in both risk groups.

2. Causes of death. In the second HIV example, we want to know how mortality from different causes has changed after the introduction of cART and to what extent it differs in individuals with HCV coinfection. We do not want to perform a marginal analysis with AIDS-related mortality as the event, which would quantify the effect of cART on AIDS-related mortality in a hypothetical world in which individuals cannot die of anything else. Moreover, the Kaplan-Meier curve would not give an unbiased estimate because AIDS-related mortality and some other causes of mortality are not independent mechanisms.

We want to quantify the effect of cART on the different causes of death in the real world in which individuals can also die of another cause. How this is performed is one of the main topics in this book. We will see that there are two effects that are of interest. One is the etiologic effect of cART on the other causes of death. Is cardiovascular mortality increased in the cART era due to the side effects of cART? But even if cART has no direct effect on the other causes, there may be an indirect effect because individuals that no longer die of AIDS will ultimately die of something else. We return to these issues in Chapters 4 and 5. The main conclusions are summarized in Chapter 6.

3. SI as intermediate event. In the third HIV example, we perform a competing risks analysis if we want to quantify the distribution of time from HIV infection to either the SI switch or AIDS as the first event.

The SI switch is not lethal, and progression to AIDS and death can also occur after the switch to SI. Similarly, an SI switch can also occur after AIDS diagnosis. We can study the time from AIDS diagnosis to death. Then we choose AIDS diagnosis instead of HIV infection as time origin. If we want to quantify the effect of the SI switch after AIDS diagnosis on progression to death, we can perform a classical survival analysis with death as the end point and SI as a time-varying covariable (see Section 4.5.3). An alternative approach is to use an illness-death multi-state model. In a multi-state model, the SI state plays a dual role. It not only acts as a time-varying covariable; it is also an intermediate state that one can enter and leave, and we can quantify the probability to be in the SI state at any point in time (see Section 4.5.3). We can also specify a more general multi-state model in which SI and AIDS are seen as intermediate states in the process from HIV infection to death (see Chapter 3, Section 4.5 and Section 5.2.2).

If we combine states, the type of analysis changes. If we study time from HIV infection to overall mortality, ignoring the intermediate events, we perform an overall survival analysis. If pre-AIDS mortality is absent in our data or if it can be assumed to be non-informative for AIDS, we can also estimate the marginal distribution of time from HIV infection to AIDS. Both are performed using techniques from classical survival analysis.

1.6.3 Bone marrow transplantation

The type of study question in the computer practicals is adapted to the topics that are explained in the respective chapter. In Section 1.12 we use techniques from classical survival analysis to quantify event-free survival and the effect of EBMT risk score. In Section 2.10 we split both event types and use a competing risks analysis to estimate the distribution of time to relapse and time to relapse-free mortality. We test whether the distributions differ by value of EBMT risk score. In Section 3.8 we use a multi-state model to estimate the transition probabilities between the different states. In Section 4.10 we quantify the effect of EBMT risk score on the three transition hazards via a proportional hazards regression model. We also investigate whether the effect of a relapse on mortality has changed over time. In Section 5.8 we use results from this regression model to quantify effects on the cumulative probability.

1.7 Notation

In this section we introduce the framework and our notation for the competing risks setting. For multi-state models they are introduced in Section 3.2.

The random variable that represents the event time, of any type, is denoted by T and the type of event is denoted by E. We use words like "AIDS" and "SI" to describe event types, but we also use numbers $1, 2, \ldots, K$, with K representing the total number of competing risks. The time until the occurrence of an event of type k is described by the random variable T_k. If a competing event happens, the event of type k will never happen; mathematically we say that the event of type k happens at time infinity. Hence we have

$$T_k = \begin{cases} T & \text{if } E = k \\ \infty & \text{if } E \neq k \end{cases} \tag{1.1}$$

If interest is in one specific type of end point, we can combine all other event types and assume $K = 2$. Then, the time to any of the competing events is described by a random variable T°. It has the value ∞ if the event of interest occurs and has the value T otherwise. If $K = 1$ we are in the classical survival setting with only one event type.

The distribution of T is described by the overall cumulative incidence function F: $F(t) = P(T \leq t)$; we write $T \sim F$. The distribution of T_k is described by the cause-specific cumulative incidence function F_k; $T_k \sim F_k$

and we have
$$F_k(t) = P(T_k \le t) = P(T \le t, E = k).$$

We use a bar to describe the complement of a cumulative event probability: $\overline{F_k} = 1 - F_k$ and $\overline{F} = 1 - F$. Note that $\overline{F}(t)$ is the overall survival function $P(T > t)$.

The hazard corresponding to F, the overall hazard, is denoted by h, and h_k is the subdistribution hazard corresponding to F_k. The cause-specific hazard for cause k is denoted by λ_k. We use a Greek letter to emphasize that the cause-specific hazard does not have a one-to-one relation with some cause-specific cumulative incidence (see Section 2.2.1).

In the data set there may be right censoring for reasons other than competing risks, as well as left truncation due to late entry. Let C represent time to censoring, not due to a competing risk. We observe $X = \min(T, C)$, the minimum of T and C. We also know which time occurred first, which is denoted via the indicator Δ:
$$\Delta = \begin{cases} 1 & \text{if } T < C \\ 0 & \text{if } C < T \end{cases}$$

The time at which an individual comes under observation is represented by V. The time X is observed only if $X > V$. If there is no late entry, V is zero for all individuals. It is useful to attach a probability distribution to the censoring and entry times. We write $C \sim \Gamma$, hence $\Gamma(t) = P(C \le t)$, and $V \sim \Phi$, i.e. $\Phi(t) = P(V \le t)$.

The observed data is represented as $\{(v_1, x_1, e_1\delta_1), \ldots, (v_N, x_N, e_N\delta_N)\}$, where N is the sample size. We use $t_{(1)} < t_{(2)} < \ldots < t_{(n)}$ to denote the ordered distinct observed event times. Note that $n < N$ if some individuals have the same observed event time. Similarly we let $c_{(1)} < \ldots < c_{(n_c)}$ and $v_{(1)} < \ldots < v_{(n_l)}$ denote the ordered distinct observed censoring and entry times respectively. Let m_i be the number of censorings at $c_{(i)}$, and let w_i be the number of entries at $v_{(i)}$. Entries, censorings and events may occur at the same time point. In that case we assume the ordering $t_{(i)} < c_{(j)} < v_{(j')}$.

For each $t_{(i)}$, define $d_k(t_{(i)})$ as the number of observed events of type k at $t_{(i)}$ and $d(t_{(i)})$ as the number of observed events of any type at $t_{(i)}$. We make a distinction between individuals that are "observed to be at risk" and those that are "in the risk set" as well as between "censoring" and "leaving the risk set". This distinction is necessary for estimation of the subdistribution hazard. Individuals that are censored due to a competing event remain in the risk set, even though they are no longer at risk for experiencing the event of interest (see Section 2.4). Although conceptually a different mechanism, the correction for left truncation is similar to the way right censored data are incorporated: an individual is included while he is observed to be at risk. Let $R(t)$ denote the group of individuals that are observed to be at risk at time t. Let $r(t)$ be the number of individuals that is observed and event free at time t. Hence, $r(t)$ is the size of $R(t)$: $r(t) = \#R(t) = \#\{i \mid x_i \ge t \wedge v_i \le t\}$. We use $r^*(t)$ to denote the extended number at risk at t, which also includes individuals that had an earlier competing event.

We assume that every individual experiences at most one event type. If an individual experiences multiple competing event types at the same time, this is usually a consequence of incomplete information. In reality both events occurred somewhat earlier and at unequal time points, but they were observed to have happened at the same time. Some approaches have been suggested to analyse such tied event types [99].

We make a distinction between variable and covariable. We use the word variable as long as we talk about some characteristic of an individual. When it is included in a regression model it is called a covariable. The covariables for individual i are denoted by the vector $\mathbf{Z}_i = (Z_{i1}, \ldots, Z_{ip})^\top$. The parameters that quantify the effect of the covariables in a regression model are described by the vector $\boldsymbol{\beta}^\top = (\beta_1, \ldots, \beta_p)$. We use $\boldsymbol{\beta}^\top \mathbf{Z}_i$ as a shorthand notation for the score $\sum_{k=1}^p \beta_k \times Z_{ik}$.

We use the shorthand notations "$\sum$" and "$\prod$" for sum and product. Hence, if $a_1, \ldots, a_m$ is a sequence of numbers, then $\sum a_i = a_1 + a_2 + \ldots + a_m$ and $\prod a_i = a_1 \times a_2 \times \ldots \times a_m$.

1.8 Basic techniques from survival analysis

We formally define the main concepts and give a summary of the most important results from classical survival analysis, i.e. the situation in which competing events are absent or treated as censored observations. We use T to represent the event time.

1.8.1 Main concepts and theoretical relations

The definitions differ slightly depending on whether the distribution of T is discrete or continuous.

The distribution of T is discrete if events can only occur at a limited number of time points, say at $\mathcal{T} = \{t_1, \ldots, t_L\}$. Then the hazard at time $t_l \in \mathcal{T}$ is defined as the conditional probability of having an event at t_l, given that the individual was still event-free just before t_l. There are different ways to denote that an individual was still event-free just before time t_l; we can write "$T \geq t_l$", "$T > t_{l-1}$" or "$T > t_l-$". We have

$$h(t_l) = P(T = t_l \mid T \geq t_l) = P(T = t_l \mid T > t_{l-1}) = P(T = t_l \mid T > t_l-)$$
$$= \frac{F(t_l) - F(t_{l-1})}{\overline{F}(t_{l-1})}. \tag{1.2}$$

From the last line we see that the hazard is uniquely determined by F. We also see that the probability to have an event at time t_l is

$$P(T = t_l) = F(t_l) - F(t_{l-1})$$
$$= \overline{F}(t_{l-1}) \times h(t_l). \tag{1.3}$$

The cumulative hazard is defined as the sum of the hazards

$$H(t) = \sum_{t_l \leq t} h(t_l). \tag{1.4}$$

It is a non-decreasing function that can be defined for any time point t but only changes value at $t_l \in \mathcal{T}$. It has the value zero until t_1.

The hazard is uniquely determined by F, but the same holds in reverse:

$$\overline{F}(t) = P(T > t) = \prod_{t_l \leq t} \{1 - h(t_l)\}. \tag{1.5}$$

This property is the basis for the Kaplan-Meier estimator as well as the product-limit form of the estimator of the cause-specific cumulative incidence. We explain how it is derived.

We write the probability $P(T > t)$ as a product of conditional probabilities. For $t > s$ we have

$$P(T > t \mid T > s) = \frac{P(T > t \text{ and } T > s)}{P(T > s)} = \frac{P(T > t)}{P(T > s)}.$$

Hence, the probability of remaining event-free beyond t, $P(T > t)$, is the product of the probability of remaining event-free beyond s and the conditional probability of remaining event-free beyond t given that one was event-free until s: $P(T > s) \times P(T > t \mid T > s)$. Applying this rule repeatedly over the event times $t_1, t_2, \ldots$ until the last one before t, we obtain[10]

$$P(T > t) = P(T > t_1) \times P(T > t_2 \mid T > t_1) \times \ldots$$
$$= \prod_{t_l \leq t} P(T > t_l \mid T > t_{l-1}) \tag{1.6}$$

Relation (1.5) follows because

$$P(T > t_l \mid T > t_{l-1}) = 1 - P(T = t_l \mid T > t_{l-1}) = 1 - h(t_l).$$

The distribution of T is continuous if T can take any value over some time range. The hazard at time t is defined as the conditional probability of an event in a tiny interval from t to $t + \Delta t$, given that the individual is still at risk at the beginning of that interval, divided by the length of the interval.

---

[10]The second line includes $P(T > t_1 \mid T > t_0)$. We define t_0 as some time point before t_1, e.g. $t_0 = 0$, such that $P(T > t_1 \mid T > t_0) = P(T > t_1)$.

Formally we write

$$h(t) = \lim_{\Delta t \downarrow 0} \frac{\mathrm{P}(t \le T < t + \Delta t \mid T \ge t)}{\Delta t}. \tag{1.7}$$

The hazard is uniquely determined by F via the relation

$$h(t) = \lim_{\Delta t \downarrow 0} \frac{1}{\Delta t} \frac{\overline{F}(t) - \overline{F}(t + \Delta t)}{\overline{F}(t)}$$

$$= \frac{1}{\overline{F}(t)} \lim_{\Delta t \downarrow 0} \frac{\overline{F}(t) - \overline{F}(t + \Delta t)}{\Delta t}$$

$$= -\frac{d \log \overline{F}(t)}{dt}.$$

The probability $\mathrm{P}(T = t)$ that the event happens exactly at some time t is zero. Therefore, it is replaced by the density $f(t)$. Similar to (1.3), the following relation holds:

$$f(t) = \overline{F}(t-)h(t).$$

With continuous distributions, sums change into integrals. The cumulative hazard is defined as

$$H(t) = \int_0^t h(s)ds. \tag{1.8}$$

The hazard uniquely determines the cumulative incidence via

$$\overline{F}(t) = \mathrm{P}(T > t) = \exp\{-H(t)\}. \tag{1.9}$$

1.8.2   The Kaplan-Meier product-limit estimator

The Kaplan-Meier estimator is the nonparametric estimator of the survival function in the presence of right censored and left truncated data. With a nonparametric estimator we make no assumptions with respect to the structure of the distribution. We do not assume that the event time data come from some parametric distribution like the Weibull or log-normal. A nonparametric estimator treats the data "as is": the data comes from a discrete distribution in which events can only occur at the observed event times, irrespective of whether the true distribution is discrete or continuous. Therefore, we estimate $\overline{F}$ using the hazard-based product property for a discrete distribution (1.5).

We estimate the hazard at the observed event times. Under the assumption of non-informative right censoring and left truncation, subjects that are under observation at time t represent all subjects that are event-free just before t, including the unobserved ones. Then $h(t_{(i)})$ can be estimated by the observed proportion that has an event at $t_{(i)}$,

$$\widehat{h}(t_{(i)}) = \frac{d(t_{(i)})}{r(t_{(i)})}. \tag{1.10}$$

The Kaplan-Meier estimator follows

$$\widehat{F}^{\text{PL}}(t) = \prod_{t_{(j)} \leq t} \left\{ 1 - \frac{d(t_{(j)})}{r(t_{(j)})} \right\}. \tag{1.11}$$

In this book, we use the superscript PL for estimators that have a "product-limit" structure[11]. The reason for "product" is clear by now. The term "limit" comes from its behaviour when the observed event times come from a continuous distribution. If the sample size increases, the number of distinct observed event times increases as well, but the product-limit formula still holds. With sample size infinity, the Kaplan-Meier estimate is equivalent to the estimator that is based on equation (1.9)[12]

$$\widehat{F}^*(t) = \exp\left\{ -\widehat{H}(t) \right\}, \tag{1.12}$$

with the cumulative hazard estimated via

$$\widehat{H}(t) = \sum_{t_{(j)} \leq t} \widehat{h}(t_{(j)}) = \sum_{t_{(j)} \leq t} \frac{d(t_{(j)})}{r(t_{(j)})}. \tag{1.13}$$

$\widehat{H}(t)$ is called the Nelson-Aalen estimator of the cumulative hazard.

With completely observed event time data, i.e. if there is no right censoring nor left truncation, the Kaplan-Meier estimator has an equivalent formulation as a cumulative frequency of observed events

$$\widehat{F}^{\text{EC}}(t) = \frac{\sum_{t_{(j)} \leq t} d(t_{(j)})}{N}. \tag{1.14}$$

This type of estimator, which directly calculates the cumulative fraction of events, is called the empirical cumulative distribution function (ECDF) and we use the superscript EC.

The reason for the equivalence is that individuals leave the risk set only when events happen, which implies $r(t_{(j+1)}) = r(t_{(j)}) - d(t_{(j)})$. As a consequence, for two subsequent event times $t_{(j)}$ and $t_{(j+1)}$ we have

$$\left\{ 1 - \frac{d(t_{(j)})}{r(t_{(j)})} \right\} \times \left\{ 1 - \frac{d(t_{(j+1)})}{r(t_{(j+1)})} \right\} = \left\{ \frac{r(t_{(j+1)})}{r(t_{(j)})} \right\} \times \left\{ \frac{r(t_{(j+1)}) - d(t_{(j+1)})}{r(t_{(j+1)})} \right\}$$

$$= \frac{r(t_{(j+1)}) - d(t_{(j+1)})}{r(t_{(j)})}.$$

Repeating this from the first event time $t_{(1)}$ until the last event time $t_{(i)}$ before t, we end up with

$$\prod_{j=1}^{i} \left\{ 1 - \frac{d(t_{(j)})}{r(t_{(j)})} \right\} = \frac{r(t_{(i)}) - d(t_{(i)})}{N} = \frac{N - \sum_{t_{(j)} \leq t} d(t_{(j)})}{N},$$

---

[11]The Kaplan-Meier is often called the product-limit estimator.
[12]This is usually called the Fleming-Harrington estimator.

which establishes the equivalence. The last equality follows because $r(t_{(i)}) - d(t_{(i)})$ is the number of individuals without an event until t.

With right censored and left truncated data, the Kaplan-Meier is equivalent to a weighted ECDF form. A similar equivalence holds in the competing risks setting (see Section 2.4.3.1).

1.8.2.1 Confidence intervals

Confidence intervals around the Kaplan-Meier estmator of the survival function can be constructed in several ways. We write "var" for the variance and "s.e." for its square root, the standard error. Let k_α be the $1 - \alpha/2$ quantile of the standard normal distribution. We leave out the explicit reference to the Kaplan-Meier via the subscript PL and write $\widehat{\overline{F}}$.

The variance of the Kaplan-Meier estimator is best estimated via the variance of the Nelson-Aalen estimator of the cumulative hazard (1.13). The most commonly used are the Aalen estimator and the Greenwood estimator, which have the following forms:

$$\text{Aalen:} \quad \widehat{\text{var}}\left\{\widehat{H}(t)\right\} = \sum_{t_{(j)} \leq t} \frac{d(t_{(j)})}{r^2(t_{(j)})} \tag{1.15}$$

$$\text{Greenwood:} \quad \widehat{\text{var}}\left\{\widehat{H}(t)\right\} = \sum_{t_{(j)} \leq t} \frac{d(t_{(j)})}{r(t_{(j)})\{r(t_{(j)}) - d(t_{(j)})\}} \tag{1.16}$$

Using $\widehat{\overline{F}}(t) \approx \exp\{-\widehat{H}(t)\}$ (see (1.12)) and the delta method[13], we obtain as variance estimator of the Kaplan-Meier

$$\widehat{\text{var}}\left\{\widehat{\overline{F}}(t)\right\} = \left\{\widehat{\overline{F}}(t)\right\}^2 \times \widehat{\text{var}}\left\{\widehat{H}(t)\right\}. \tag{1.17}$$

The Aalen form is preferred when estimating the variance of the cumulative hazard, whereas the Greenwood form has been shown to perform better when estimating the variance of the survival function [54].

The most straightforward $(1 - \alpha) \times 100\%$ confidence interval around the estimated survival function is on the "plain" or "linear" scale

$$\widehat{\overline{F}}(t) \pm k_\alpha \, \widehat{\text{s.e.}}\left\{\widehat{\overline{F}}(t)\right\} = \widehat{\overline{F}}(t) \pm k_\alpha \, \widehat{\overline{F}}(t) \times \widehat{\text{s.e.}}\left\{\widehat{H}(t)\right\}. \tag{1.18}$$

It may yield values below 0 and above 1 and is not recommended [100, p.17].

A better approach is to first calculate the $(1-\alpha) \times 100\%$ confidence interval around the Nelson-Aalen estimator of the cumulative hazard

$$\widehat{H}(t) \pm k_\alpha \, \widehat{\text{s.e.}}\left\{\widehat{H}(t)\right\}.$$

---

[13]$\text{var}\{f(X)\} = \{f'(X)\}^2 \times \text{var}(X)$ with $f(X) = \exp(-X)$

We use the relation $\widehat{H}(t) \approx -\log\{\widehat{\overline{F}}(t)\}$ to obtain

$$\exp\left[\log\{\widehat{\overline{F}}(t)\} \pm k_\alpha \, \widehat{\text{s.e.}}\{\widehat{H}(t)\}\right] = \widehat{\overline{F}}(t) \times \exp\left[\pm k_\alpha \, \widehat{\text{s.e.}}\{\widehat{H}(t)\}\right]. \quad (1.19)$$

Using (1.17) this can be rewritten as

$$\widehat{\overline{F}}(t) \times \exp\left[\frac{\pm k_\alpha \, \widehat{\text{s.e.}}\{\widehat{\overline{F}}(t)\}}{\widehat{\overline{F}}(t)}\right]. \quad (1.20)$$

This scale is commonly called the "log" scale and has been recommended for most situations [100, p.17]. It can attain values above 1, but never below 0..

An alternative form, which is guaranteed to give confidence intervals between 0 and 1, first calculates the confidence interval around the logarithm of the cumulative hazard

$$\log \widehat{H}(t) \pm k_\alpha \, \widehat{\text{s.e.}}\left\{\log \widehat{H}(t)\right\}.$$

Using $\log\{-\log \widehat{\overline{F}}(t)\} \approx \log \widehat{H}(t)$, we transform it back to a confidence interval around the estimated survival function. We obtain the form a^b, with

$$a = \widehat{\overline{F}}(t)$$

$$b = \exp\left[\pm k_\alpha \, \widehat{\text{s.e.}}\left\{\log \widehat{H}(t)\right\}\right]. \quad (1.21)$$

Using the delta method, $\widehat{H}(t) \approx -\log\{\widehat{\overline{F}}(t)\}$ and (1.17), we derive

$$\widehat{\text{s.e.}}\left\{\log \widehat{H}(t)\right\} = \frac{\widehat{\text{s.e.}}\left\{\widehat{H}(t)\right\}}{\widehat{H}(t)} = \frac{\widehat{\text{s.e.}}\left\{\widehat{\overline{F}}(t)\right\}}{-\widehat{\overline{F}}(t)\log\{\widehat{\overline{F}}(t)\}}. \quad (1.22)$$

Because of the relation $\log\{\widehat{H}(t)\} \approx \log\{-\log \widehat{\overline{F}}(t)\}$, it is called the "log-log" or "complementary log-log" scale, abbreviated as "cloglog". It has been shown to perform well even in small samples with heavy censoring ($N \approx 25$ with up to 50% censoring, [15]).

Expression (1.20) and the last term in (1.22) don't make any reference to a hazard and can also be used in competing risks and multi-state settings.

We gave expressions for the confidence interval around the estimate of the survival function. If we want to calculate the confidence intervals around the estimate of the cumulative incidence, we can first calculate the confidence interval around $\widehat{\overline{F}}$ and use $y = 1 - (1 - y)$. However, we can also construct confidence intervals directly around $\widehat{F}$, applying the delta method for the log and log-log transformations. We then obtain the following expressions:

$$\text{linear scale: } \widehat{F}(t) \pm k_\alpha \, \widehat{s.e.}\Big\{\widehat{F}(t)\Big\}$$

$$\text{log scale: } \widehat{F}(t) \times \exp\left\{\frac{\pm k_\alpha \, \widehat{s.e.}\big\{\widehat{F}(t)\big\}}{\widehat{F}(t)}\right\}$$

$$\text{log-log scale: } a = \widehat{F}(t)$$

$$b = \exp\left[\frac{\pm k_\alpha \, \widehat{s.e.}\big\{\widehat{F}(t)\big\}}{\widehat{F}(t)\log\big\{\widehat{F}(t)\big\}}\right] \tag{1.23}$$

Note that $\widehat{s.e.}\{\widehat{F}(t)\} = \widehat{s.e.}\{\widehat{F}(t)\}$. These expressions have mainly been used in competing risks and multi-state settings. When software refers to the log or log-log scale, it is important to know whether it refers to (1.20) and (1.21) or the ones in (1.23).

1.8.3   Nonparametric group comparisons

If we want to determine whether the time-to-event distributions of two or more groups are different, the log-rank test is most commonly used. It can be seen as one member of a family of tests with similar structure. They all test for a difference in hazards over time between groups, but they differ in the weight that is given to different parts of the time scale.

These tests compare the observed number of events per group with the expected number under the null hypothesis that the groups have the same event time distribution. For each group g and time $t_{(j)}$, let $d^{(g)}(t_{(j)})$ be the number of observed events in g and let $r^{(g)}(t_{(j)})$ be the number of individuals in g that is at risk at $t_{(j)}$. The expected number under the null hypothesis is estimated as the observed overall proportion that has an event at $t_{(j)}$, $d(t_{(j)})/r(t_{(j)})$, multiplied by the observed number at risk in group g. For two groups, the test is based on the comparison within one group only, say $g = 1$. The comparison for the other group is completely determined by the first because $d^{(2)}(t_{(j)}) = d(t_{(j)}) - d^{(1)}(t_{(j)})$. The form of the test statistic Z is

$$Z = \sum_{j=1}^{n} W(t_{(j)})\left\{d^{(1)}(t_{(j)}) - r^{(1)}(t_{(j)})\frac{d(t_{(j)})}{r(t_{(j)})}\right\}. \tag{1.24}$$

$W(t_{(j)})$ is a weight function; if it is chosen to be equal to one, the log-rank test is obtained. Rewriting the statistic we see that it is based on a comparison of the estimate of the group specific hazard and the hazard estimate if all groups are combined:

$$Z = \sum_{j=1}^{n} W(t_{(j)})r^{(1)}(t_{(j)})\left\{\frac{d^{(1)}(t_{(j)})}{r^{(1)}(t_{(j)})} - \frac{d(t_{(j)})}{r(t_{(j)})}\right\}. \tag{1.25}$$

This is equivalent to a weighted difference between the group-specific estimates of the hazard:

$$Z = \sum_{j=1}^{n} W(t_{(j)}) \frac{r^{(1)}(t_{(j)})r^{(2)}(t_{(j)})}{r^{(1)}(t_{(j)}) + r^{(2)}(t_{(j)})} \left[\frac{d^{(1)}(t_{(j)})}{r^{(1)}(t_{(j)})} - \frac{d^{(2)}(t_{(j)})}{r^{(2)}(t_{(j)})} \right] . \qquad (1.26)$$

When comparing more than two groups, the test statistic becomes more complicated but the basic idea remains the same.

Inference is based on the standardized statistic $Z/\mathrm{var}(Z)$. Under the null hypothesis of no difference between the groups, and if the sample size goes to infinity, it has a chi-squared distribution with number of degrees of freedom equal to the number of groups minus one. The log-rank test is equivalent to the score test from a Cox proportional hazards model that uses group membership as single covariable.

These tests are not very powerful when effects are non-proportional on the hazard. Therefore, other tests that already existed for completely observed data have been extended to the setting of right censored survival data[14]. Examples are the Kolmogorov-Smirnov test and the adaptive Neyman's smooth test [62]. So far they have not been used very often.

1.8.4 Cox proportional hazards model

If we want to quantify the effect of covariables on the event time distribution, we define a regression model. Several types of models can be formulated. Accelerated failure time models are specified through parameters that quantify effects on the event time. They are usually fully parametric models, in which the event time distribution is assumed to have a specific form like Weibull or log-normal. They resemble standard linear regression models.

Another approach is to use a model in which parameters quantify effects on the hazard or the cumulative incidence. A common choice is to specify a semiparametric model. In such a model, the effect of the covariables is quantified via parameters, but is assumed constant over time. A nonparametric specification is used for the trend over time. The Cox proportional hazards model is the most well-known example.

In the Cox model, parameters quantify effects on the hazard. In its simplest form, the hazard for a subject i with covariable values $\mathbf{Z}_i$ is described via

$$h(t \mid \mathbf{Z}_i) = h_0(t) \exp(\boldsymbol{\beta}^\top \mathbf{Z}_i) . \qquad (1.27)$$

When comparing two individuals with covariable values $\mathbf{Z}_j$ and $\mathbf{Z}_i$ via the relative hazard $h(t \mid \mathbf{Z}_j)/h(t \mid \mathbf{Z}_i)$ we obtain

$$\frac{h(t \mid \mathbf{Z}_j)}{h(t \mid \mathbf{Z}_i)} = \frac{h_0(t) \exp(\boldsymbol{\beta}^\top \mathbf{Z}_j)}{h_0(t) \exp(\boldsymbol{\beta}^\top \mathbf{Z}_i)} = \exp\{\boldsymbol{\beta}^\top (\mathbf{Z}_j - \mathbf{Z}_i)\} .$$

---

[14]The extension to left truncated data is possible as well.

The parameter vector $\boldsymbol{\beta}$ is estimated by maximizing the partial likelihood. We assume that all event times are distinct. A number of methods exist to deal with tied event times. The most commonly used are the Breslow approximation, the Efron approximation and the exact method. We do not explain them. Given that there is an event observed at $t_{(i)}$, the conditional probability that it is from individual l is equal to

$$\frac{h_0(t_{(i)})\exp(\boldsymbol{\beta}^\top \mathbf{Z}_l)}{\sum_{j \in R(t_{(i)})} h_0(t_{(i)})\exp(\boldsymbol{\beta}^\top \mathbf{Z}_j)} = \frac{\exp(\boldsymbol{\beta}^\top \mathbf{Z}_l)}{\sum_{j \in R(t_{(i)})} \exp(\boldsymbol{\beta}^\top \mathbf{Z}_j)}.$$

The partial likelihood is the product of this expression over the observed event times. We use a slightly different, but equivalent notation that extends to the proportional subdistribution hazards model in Section 5.3. We define an "at-risk" function $\psi(t)$ as

$$\psi_l(t) = \begin{cases} 0 & \text{if person } l \text{ not at risk at } t \\ 1 & \text{if person } l \text{ is at risk at } t \end{cases} \tag{1.28}$$

The partial likelihood can be written as

$$L(\boldsymbol{\beta}) = \prod_{\substack{i=1 \\ \delta_i=1}}^{N} \left\{ \frac{\psi_i(t_i)\exp(\boldsymbol{\beta}^\top \mathbf{Z}_i)}{\sum_{j=1}^{N} \psi_j(t_i)\exp(\boldsymbol{\beta}^\top \mathbf{Z}_j)} \right\}. \tag{1.29}$$

Note that for the censored individuals the term has value one. Since the effect of the covariables does not depend on time, the actual event times can be ignored when estimating the parameters. Only the ordering of the event times matters because it determines the risk sets in the denominator.

Since the hazard is an instantaneous quantity, we can also quantify the effect of a covariable that varies over time. We call this a time-varying co-variable; alternative names are time-updated covariable and time-dependent covariable. Variables that change over time can be classified as internal or external [51]. An internal time-varying variable is a characteristic that develops over time as a consequence of some mechanism within the unit of investigation. In the life sciences, the typical example is a marker of disease progression. Its development is non-deterministic and stops when the person dies. An external time-varying variable is a characteristic that changes over time in a more or less independent way. For external time-varying variables, a distinction can be made between defined and ancillary ones. A defined time-varying variable changes in a deterministic way; for each individual in the study its value is already known at his time origin. Examples are age and calendar time of follow-up. An ancillary time-varying variable is an external characteristic that changes in a non-deterministic way. An example is air-pollution. Although individuals in the study may contribute to its value, it is not linked at the individual level and can also be measured after individuals in the study have died.

Results from a Cox model can be used to quantify effects on the cumulative scale, both for individuals in the sample as well as for new individuals. For this, we need an estimate of the baseline hazard. Breslow's estimate is most commonly used; it is defined as

$$\widehat{H}_0(t) = \sum_{t_{(j)} \leq t} \frac{1}{\sum_{l=1}^{N} \psi_l(t_{(j)}) \exp(\widehat{\boldsymbol{\beta}}^\top \mathbf{Z}_l)} . \tag{1.30}$$

If the covariables do not change over time, then we use (1.9) to obtain an estimate of the survival curve for an individual l

$$\begin{aligned}
\widehat{\overline{F}}(t|\mathbf{Z}_l) &= \exp\left\{ -\int_0^t \widehat{h}_0(s) \exp(\widehat{\boldsymbol{\beta}}^\top \mathbf{Z}_l) ds \right\} \\
&= \exp\left\{ -\widehat{H}_0(t) e^{\widehat{\boldsymbol{\beta}}^\top \mathbf{Z}_l} \right\} \tag{1.31} \\
&= \widehat{\overline{F}}_0(t)^{\exp(\widehat{\boldsymbol{\beta}}^\top \mathbf{Z}_l)} .
\end{aligned}$$

$\widehat{\overline{F}}_0(t) = \exp\{ -\widehat{H}_0(t) \}$ is the estimated survival curve if $\widehat{\boldsymbol{\beta}}^\top \mathbf{Z}_l = 0$, i.e. for an individual that has the value "zero" for all covariables. Often, covariables are centered by the statistical program, such that the baseline hazard describes the hazard for an "average individual". Numeric variables are typically centered at the mean or median value. For a categorical variable the most frequent value is often chosen as reference, but a mixture of values according to the frequency distribution is another option, e.g. 60% male and 40% female[15]. The choice of reference value affects the value of the baseline hazard, but it does not affect the shape of the baseline hazard and the individual predictions.

If the model includes a time-varying covariable, then quantification of effects on the cumulative scale becomes more difficult. In Formula (1.31), we can no longer split the baseline hazard and the effect of the covariable, because both depend on time. Furthermore, we need to know how the variable changes over time. For a defined external time-varying covariable, the change is deterministic. For an ancillary one we only need to know how it develops at the population level; during the period of observation this is observed. For an internal time-varying covariable, we additionally need a model for its development.

We can use the scaled Schoenfeld residuals to test for proportionality. The scaled Schoenfeld residual s_{il}^* is defined for each parameter l and at each event time $t_{(i)}$. Its expected value is $E(s_{il}^*) = \beta_l(t_{(i)})$. Proportionality is tested against deviations of the form $\beta_l(t) = \beta_l + \theta_l f(t)$, with $f(t)$ a function of time that is chosen by the user. The null hypothesis $H_0 : \theta_l = 0$ corresponds to proportionality. In case of non-proportionality, the function $f(t)$ allows us to get an idea of the time trend. We make a scatterplot of s_{il}^* against $f(t_{(i)})$ and fit a smooth line through the points. If the effect is proportional, then the line

---

[15]See the help file for the `survfit.coxph` function in R for a discussion on using the mean value.

must be approximately horizontal; if we see a more or less straight line, then the effect changes over time according to the function $f(t)$.

If we have a categorical variable for which the effect is not proportional, we can use a stratified Cox model that allows for a separate baseline hazard per value g of that variable:

$$h_g(t \mid \mathbf{Z}_i) = h_{g,0}(t) \, \exp(\boldsymbol{\beta}^\top \mathbf{Z}_i) \,.$$

Parameter estimation in a stratified Cox model is performed by maximizing the product of the stratum specific partial likelihoods

$$L(\boldsymbol{\beta}) = \prod_{g \in \mathcal{G}} L^g(\boldsymbol{\beta}) \,, \tag{1.32}$$

where $L^g(\boldsymbol{\beta})$ is the partial likelihood (1.29) evaluated over the individuals that belong to stratum g. If the parameters $\boldsymbol{\beta}$ are allowed to differ per strata, then the terms $L^g(\boldsymbol{\beta}_g)$ in the product have nothing in common and fitting such a stratified Cox model boils down to fitting separate Cox models per stratum.

Another semi-parametric model is the proportional odds model. In this model, covariable effects are modeled on the cumulative incidence via

$$\text{logit}\{P(T \le t \mid \mathbf{Z}_i)\} = \alpha_0(t) + \boldsymbol{\beta}^\top \mathbf{Z}_i \,, \tag{1.33}$$

or equivalently

$$\frac{P(T \le t \mid \mathbf{Z}_i)}{1 - P(T \le t \mid \mathbf{Z}_i)} = \pi_0(t) \, \exp(\boldsymbol{\beta}^\top \mathbf{Z}_i) \,. \tag{1.34}$$

Note the similarity in structure to the proportional hazards model. Effects are assumed constant over time on the scale of the odds of the cumulative incidence. $\pi_0(t) = \exp\{\alpha(t)\}$ is the baseline odds, the odds when all covariables are equal to the reference value. At a fixed time point, it is a logistic regression in which $T \le t$ defines the outcome. We briefly describe parameter estimation in the proportional odds model in Section 5.4.

Both the proportional odds model and the Cox proportional hazards model require the investigator to choose one time scale as the principal one. Trends over this time scale are specified via the baseline hazard or odds. Sometimes, more than one time scale is of importance. For example, childhood cancer survivors are at increased risk of hospitalization. Hospitalization rates may be determined by both age, i.e. time since birth, and time since cancer diagnosis. If we want to add a second time scale to the analysis, it can be included as covariable. A more flexible approach is to specify a Poisson regression model in which both time scales can be given equal importance [50].

1.8.5   Counting process format

For most analyses in this book, data is best presented using a format that originates from the counting process formulation of survival analysis. The counting process formulation uses notation and theory that facilitates mathematical statistical development. In the counting process format, the follow-up time of an individual is split into intervals that are determined by characteristics that change during his follow-up. These can be final events or end of follow-up, but can also be covariables that change over time, states that he enters or leaves over time or weights that vary over time.

The simplest situation in which the counting process format is useful is when we need to correct for left truncation. An individual's follow-up data is expressed by three variables instead of two: apart from the event or censoring time (`event.time`) and a variable denoting whether the event time is observed or right censored (`status`), a third variable is used that gives the time at which the individual came under observation (`entry.time`). Consider the follow-up data from three example individuals:

id	entry.time	event.time	status
1	0.0	4.3	1
2	0.0	5.6	0
3	3.4	7.7	1

The first individual experienced the event after 4.3 years, and had been in follow-up since her time origin. The second individual, who had also been in follow-up since his time origin, was censored after 5.6 years. The value 3.4 of the third individual describes that he entered the study and came under observation 3.4 years after the event that determined his time origin.

A similar way of presentation is used for time-varying variables. As an example, suppose we want to investigate whether the time from HIV infection to AIDS has changed over calendar time. Calendar time is categorized into three periods: before 1988, from 1988 to 1992 and after 1992[16]. One way of analysis is to use a fixed covariable "calendar period of HIV infection". However, individuals that became infected before 1988 and had a long follow-up also contribute to later calendar periods. An alternative approach is to use a time-varying covariable "calendar period of follow-up".

In Figure 1.17 we describe the follow-up history over calendar time for ten individuals. Solid lines denote the time from HIV infection until AIDS or censoring per individual. For example, individual 1 became infected in 1985, at 1985.7 if the year is represented numerically, and developed AIDS 8.2 years later at 1993.9. In his personal time scale, his calendar period of follow-up changed at 2.3 years and 6.3 years, and he experienced the event after 8.2 years. In the data set, his history is split over three rows:

id	start.time	stop.time	status	cal.period
1	0	2.3	0	< 1988
1	2.3	6.3	0	1988–1991
1	6.3	8.2	1	> 1991

---

[16]This more or less represents changes in the availability of antiretroviral treatment.

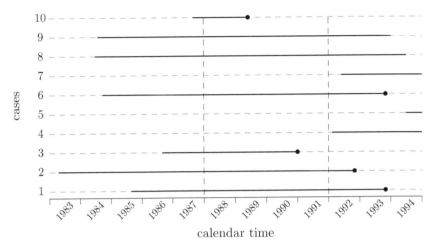

FIGURE 1.17
Follow-up data for ten example individuals. The vertical dashed lines define the three calendar periods of follow-up.

At the end of the first period, he is still event-free and the value of his status variable is zero. One can also say that he is censored for follow-up in the first period at 2.3 years. This can be seen as a form of administrative censoring, as if we were performing the analysis at the end of 1988[17]. He enters the second period at 2.3 years. This can be seen as a form of late entry that induces left truncation. He comes under observation for experiencing the event "AIDS between 1988 and 1992" at 2.3 years, whereas an individual that became infected at the same time 1985.7 but developed AIDS within 2.3 years would be missed for the second calendar time period. This has been called internal left truncation [6]. The difference with standard left truncation is that the individual that became infected and developed AIDS before 1988 has been observed. After 6.3 years, the individual is censored for the second period and he enters the third calendar period. He experiences the event during the third period at 8.2 years after HIV infection.

The basis of the representation of a time-varying variable is that every change in value generates a new row. The same structure can be used if the value of a time-varying covariable changes continuously, as is typically the case with markers of disease progression. We can see from the structure of the partial likelihood that we only need to know the values at the event times; the

---

[17]It could also be argued that it is a form of artificial censoring, which was described as a special case of competing risks (see Page 9): he remains in follow-up, but he is no longer at risk for experiencing the event "AIDS before 1988". However, the criterion for censoring holds uniformly for all individuals and the censoring time is known, also if the event happens first. This is typical for administrative censoring. See also the discussion on Page 75.

values in-between event times are not relevant. If they are not observed at all event times, we need to make assumptions with respect to their values. For example, we can use the fitted values based on a model for its developemnt over time.

Although follow-up of individuals may be spread over several rows, standard errors of the parameter estimates do not change. The essential property is that each individual has at most one event.

In Section 2.9, we see that the same data presentation can be used when individuals are included with a weight that changes over time: each line represents follow-up for a period in which the weight is constant. And in Section 4.5, a similar data presentation is used in a multi-state setting to describe the occurrence of intermediate events.

1.9   Summary and preview

Events can be seen as transitions from one state to another. When analysing time-to-event data, the event is not always observed. The event may not have happened at the end of the follow-up, which is called right censoring. And individuals may be missed altogether because they experienced the event before they would enter the study; this is called left truncation. An important requirement for unbiased estimation is that right censoring and left truncation are non-informative for the event time. We may be able to show that it is not fulfilled by using extra information, such as information on causes of death in the IDU-MSM comparison. In that case, the Kaplan-Meier can be computed, but the result is not an interpretable quantity. Non-informative censoring and truncation are assumptions that are based on our own judgement. We can argue why we think it holds, but its validity cannot be based on data.

In the classical setting, only one type of transition is considered: from some intitial state to a single final event type. If there are competing events that prevent the one of interest from occurring, we describe what would happen in the situation in which the competing events were eliminated: we want to quantify the marginal distribution. If the event of interest and the competing events are consequences of the same mechanism, the marginal distribution is often completely hypothetical. Then it is more sensible to quantify progression to the event of interest, taking account of the fact that another event type may prevent the one of interest from occurring.

This book deals with settings in which the competing types of final events are considered in their own right (competing risks analysis) and settings with intermediate events, which may be competing as well (multi-state models). Although occurrence of a competing event can be seen as a form of right censoring, this censoring is not required to be non-informative. The reason is that individuals that experience a competing event are not assumed to be represented by the ones that remain in event-free follow-up. A competing risks analysis describes progression to the different end points as they co-exist in reality.

Analysis is often based on the hazard. In a competing risks setting, two types of hazards can be defined, the cause-specific hazard and the subdistribution hazard. The cause-specific hazard is the instantaneous risk of progression to a specific type of event, conditionally on being at risk for experiencing that event; it is a rate in the classical sense. When estimating the cause-specific hazard, individuals that experience a competing event leave the risk set (Section 2.3). The subdistribution hazard is the instantaneous risk of progression to a specific type of event, conditionally on not having experienced that event. Individuals that experienced a competing event remain in the risk set. In Section 2.4.3.2, we introduce the nonparametric estimator of the subdistribution hazard. Both hazards can be used to quantify the probability to progress to a specific cause by time t, the crude risk or cause-specific cumulative incidence. The subdistribution hazard is the one that uniquely determines the crude risk; the relation between cause-specific hazard and crude risk is less straightforward.

In a multi-state model, we describe the sequence of events occurring over time. Initial events start the process, intermediate events update the state and final events terminate the follow-up. In Chapter 3 we give formal definitions and explain estimation. The basis for estimation is the transition hazard, which has the same interpretation as the cause-specific hazard. Classical survival analysis and competing risks are special cases of multi-state models.

If we want to quantify the effect of variables, we commonly use a regression model. A competing risks analysis allows us to investigate whether variables act differently on each of the event types. We concentrate on proportional hazards models. In Chapter 4 we explain modeling and estimation of effects on the cause-specific hazard and the transition hazard. In Chapter 5 we explain three ways to quantify effects on the cumulative scale of the risk.

The type of analysis, marginal, competing risks or multi-state, depends on the study objective. In the etiologic objective, we try to shed light on causal mechanisms. Another objective is prediction, either at the individual level as in a clinical setting or at the population level. In Chapter 6 we explain which type of analysis is best suited for a specific study objective.

1.10   Exercises

1. This is a simple exercise to train in the concepts of hazard, probability and cumulative incidence. We estimate the distribution of time T from birth to death for individuals in the Netherlands. Data have been downloaded from the human mortality database (`http://www.mortality.org`). For

every age a (rounded to years), the estimates of probability $P(T = a)$, hazard $P(T = a | T \geq a)$ and survival $P(T > a)$ are shown in Figure 1.18. Which line represents which quantity?

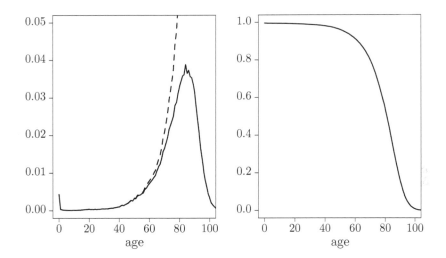

FIGURE 1.18
Mortality in Dutch population.

2. Comment on the informative censoring in this statement:

> If we want to estimate the incidence of ovarian cancer, a woman that dies of breast cancer prior to developing ovarian cancer is considered censored at her date of death. This type of censoring is informative since this patient is censored due to the occurrence of an intervening event (mortality from breast cancer).

3. We want to estimate the marginal distribution of time from bone marrow transplantation until relapse. Comment on the following statement:

> In our data, some individuals died without relapse, but they had already left the study before they died. Therefore, for relapse as end point, no competing risk of death is present in our data and the Kaplan-Meier curve is a valid estimate of the marginal distribution of time to relapse.

4. This is an exercise on how to deal with right censored data. Figure 1.19 depicts follow-up information from 1980 until 1997 on 171 HIV infected MSM that participated in the Amsterdam Cohort Studies (ACS) at the Public Health Service of Amsterdam (PHS). Each horizontal line represents one person. The solid line starts at the date of HIV infection. It ends

at January 1st, 1997 for those that were still AIDS free and in follow-up
at the PHS. The solid line can stop before 1997. It ends with a dot for
those that developed AIDS during the PHS follow-up. It ends without
a dot for those that discontinued follow-up at the PHS while still being
AIDS free. Individuals that developed AIDS after having left the PHS,
but before 1997, are represented by a dashed line from the last PHS visit
until the date of AIDS diagnosis; the dashed line ends with a dot. There
are two ways in which AIDS could be ascertained after the last PHS visit.
Either an individual developed AIDS while being followed in hospital, or
his AIDS diagnosis was found through linking with the AIDS registry.

What do we do with information from persons after they discontinued
follow-up at the PHS? Assume that nobody left the PHS because of pre-
AIDS mortality. We list five strategies:

A: **Use data as in the figure**
   Individuals without an AIDS diagnosis remain in the risk set until
   the last PHS visit (end of the solid line). We use all information
   with respect to the AIDS diagnosis. Hence, if an individual developed
   AIDS after the last PHS visit, he remains in the risk set until the date
   of diagnosis (end of the dashed line).

B: **Censor at 1-1-1997**
   We assume that all individuals without an observed AIDS diagnosis
   are still AIDS-free at 1-1-1997. They leave the risk set at that date.

C: **Only PHS follow-up**
   We do not use information with respect to AIDS diagnosis after the
   last PHS visit. Follow-up stops at the last PHS visit before 1-1-1997
   for individuals that developed AIDS later.

D: **Cutoff at 1-1-1993**
   Similar to method B, but only information until 1-1-1993 is used.

E: **Partial completion**
   If the AIDS diagnosis is less than two years after the last PHS visit,
   it is included in the analysis. AIDS-free follow-up is extended for a
   maximum of two years after the last PHS visit, but not later than
   1-1-1997.

Give your opinion on each of these strategies. For each strategy, do you
think that the Kaplan-Meier is an unbiased estimator of the distribution
of time from HIV infection to AIDS?

For each of the following pairs of strategies, we compare the Kaplan-Meier
curves. What do you expect with respect to the relative position of both?
Will one always be higher than the other?

1) A and B
2) A and C
3) B and D
4) B and E

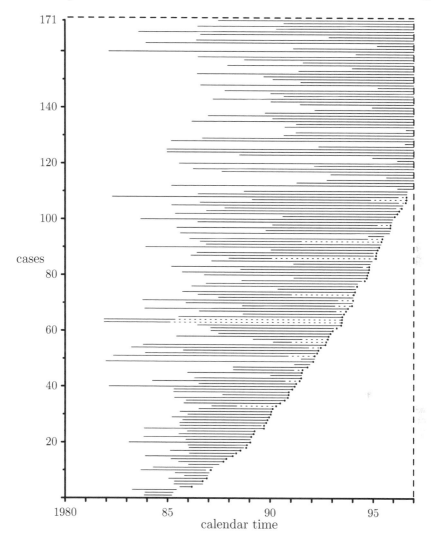

FIGURE 1.19
Graphical representation of individual follow-up of 171 MSM from the ACS.

5. Is administrative censoring informative for time to AIDS in the following situation? We want to estimate the distribution of time from HIV infection to AIDS. Individuals have been followed from HIV infection until the earliest of the event AIDS and administrative censoring on January 1st, 1996. Individuals in the study that became HIV infected in the period 1984 to 1990 were on average younger than the ones that became infected

in the period 1990 to 1996. It is known that time from HIV infection to AIDS becomes shorter with increasing age.

6. In vitro fertilization (IVF) is used as treatment for subfertility problems. The effectiveness of IVF is usually quantified via the pregnancy rate per treatment cycle. Many women discontinue treatment. It has been suggested that reported pregnancy rates in assisted reproductive technology studies are inflated due to higher dropout rates in women with a lower probability of conception.

   In a meta-analysis, observed pregnancy rate and dropout rate per cycle are compared. Each study contributes three cycles and all studies have about the same sample size. In Figure 1.20, pregnancy rates are plotted against dropout rates. A linear regression line is drawn as well.

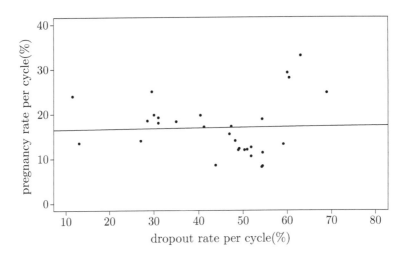

FIGURE 1.20
Relation between pregnancy rate and dropout rate per cycle.

Comment on the following statement:

> If women with a lower probability of conception were more likely to drop out, we would see higher pregnancy rates in studies with high dropout rates. The scatterplot shows no trend. Therefore, overestimation of pregnancy rates due to dropout is limited.

7. Psychiatric patients are treated in two different hospitals, A and B. We want to investigate whether the effect of the treatment on the development of side effects is the same for both hospitals. Hospital A collects information on side effects after discharge, and hospital B does not. In our analysis for hospital A we also use information after discharge, while for

hospital B we censor individuals when they are discharged. What type of distribution do we want to quantify? Under which conditions can this be a fair comparison between both hospitals?

8. This exercise is about left truncation due to late entry. We want to estimate the distribution of time from HIV infection to death, using data from a cohort study in which individuals with HIV infection are followed over time. Many individuals have been followed from HIV infection onwards, but individuals may also enter the study after HIV infection. If they do, their date of HIV infection is known.

In cohort study A, individuals had to be AIDS free in order to enter the study. In cohort study B, any HIV infected person that was alive was allowed to enter the study, also if he already developed AIDS. Individuals that died before they could enter the study are missed. We correct for left truncation effects by starting the follow-up from entry onwards. Assume that all mortality is caused by AIDS and therefore only occurs after AIDS.

With respect to the position of the late entry time relative to AIDS and death, three situations can be distinguished as described in Figure 1.21. A person in situation (I) was included in both studies. A person in situation (III) was not included in study A nor in B since he died before he could enter the study. A person in situation (II) was not included in study A, whereas in study B he was included.

Suppose there is no bias in the "full" data estimate, i.e. the estimate that

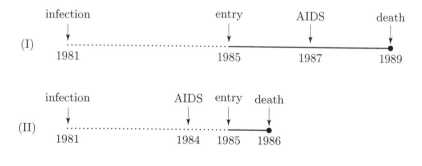

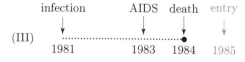

FIGURE 1.21
Three possible situations with respect to relative position of late entry, AIDS and death.

were obtained if all individuals had been followed from infection onwards. Do data from both studies give an unbiased estimate of the distribution of time from HIV infection to death? If not, which type of entry criterion leads to a biased estimate?

9.* Derive the expressions in (1.23) for the confidence intervals on the log scale and the log-log scale.

1.11   R code for classical survival analysis

We describe the standard functions in R for calculating the Kaplan-Meier curve and for fitting a Cox model[18]. These functions are contained in the survival package, which is a recommended package that comes pre-installed with the R program.

The R code in this book will be explained using the example "SI as intermediate event" from Section 1.2.2. The data set comes in two forms, which are both contained in the mstate package. In this section and in the sections on competing risks, we use the data set that is available as R object aidssi. Stata provides the same example data set for performing competing risks analyses. The other data set is available as R object aidssi2 and is used as example in the sections on multi-state models. Here we describe the aidssi data set. The contents of aidssi2 is explained in Section 3.4.1.

1.11.1   The aidssi data set

In order to access the data set in an R session, we first load the mstate package and the data set via

```
library(mstate)
data(aidssi)
```

The command library(mstate) also loads the survival package. The data contains information on two event types, "AIDS" and "SI", which compete to be the first to occur. It additionally includes information on the CCR5 genotype. Table 1.3 shows the individuals in rows 14, 3, 15 and 8. Time is given in years since HIV infection. There are two different representations of the information on the event type that occurred first. In the **cause** column, the event type is described in words, whereas in the **status** column a numeric respresentation is used. The **ccr5** column contains the information on the presence of the deletion CCR5-Δ32. Individuals that don't have the deletion have the value WW (W stands for "wild type"). Individuals that have the deletion

----

[18]All actions in R are performed via functions.

on one of the chromosomes have the value WM (M stands for "mutation")[19]. The wild type is more common: 259 individuals have WW, 65 have WM and 5 have a missing value.

TABLE 1.3
Four example individuals, `aidssi` data set

patnr	time	status	cause	ccr5
14	5.054	0	event-free	WW
3	2.234	1	AIDS	WW
15	10.196	1	AIDS	WM
8	8.605	2	SI	WW

1.11.2 Define time and status information

In general, information with respect to event and censoring is contained in two columns: one with the event/censoring time and one with the event status. In R, the `Surv` function combines both via its `time` and `event` arguments. There are three ways to specify the event status. One is to use the values "0" (for censoring) and "1" (for event). A second way is to use the logical values `FALSE` and `TRUE`, which are interpreted as "0"and "1". A third way is to use the values "1" for censoring and "2" for event.

We are interested in the combined event "AIDS or SI", i.e. in the overall cumulative incidence. Whether this event was observed can be specified using either the **status** or the **cause** variable. We use one of the logical statements

```
Surv(time=time, event=(status!=0))
Surv(time=time, event=(cause!="event-free"))
```

We can omit the argument names `time` and `event` as long as we specify the time information before the status information. The parentheses around the logical statement are not needed but are given for reasons of clarity.

When using the counting process format we specify two time columns via the `Surv` function; its argument `time` is now used to specify the entry time and the argument `time2` is used to specify the event/censoring time.

1.11.3 Perform calculations

When calculating estimates and fitting models, the R formula structure is used. In this structure, the outcome variable is specified before the $\sim$ sign and the covariables are specified after the $\sim$ sign.

With time-to-event data, the outcome is the time/event combination as combined in the `Surv` function. We calculate the Kaplan-Meier curve via the

---

[19]The data set does not contain individuals that have the CCR5-Δ32 deletion on both chromosomes. They rarely become infected with HIV.

`survfit.formula` function. If we want one Kaplan-Meier curve for the total sample, the right hand side only consists of an "intercept" 1. We assign the result to an object `KM.curve`[20].

```
KM.curve <- survfit(Surv(time, status!=0)~1, data=aidssi)
```

We fit a Cox model via the `coxph` function. If we include `ccr5` as the covariable, we write

```
fit.Cox <- coxph(Surv(time, status!=0)~ccr5, data=aidssi)
```

1.11.4   Summary of outcome

A textual summary of the result of a computation is typically obtained via the `print` or `summary` function. The latter gives more detailed information. Instead of specifying the `print` command, we can also just give the name of the object that contains the result. For example, we obtain a short summary of the Kaplan-Meier estimate by writing

```
KM.curve
```

and obtain as output

```
Call: survfit(formula = Surv(time, status != 0) ~ 1,
                                                data = aidssi)


records   n.max n.start   events  median 0.95LCL 0.95UCL
 329.00  329.00  329.00   222.00    7.30    6.44    8.36
```

For a complete numeric summary of the survival curve we use

```
summary(KM.curve)
```

Since the output is very long, we only show the first and last rows:

time	n.risk	n.event	survival	std.err	lower95%CI	upper95%CI
0.112	329	1	0.997	0.00303	0.991	1.000
0.137	328	1	0.994	0.00429	0.986	1.000
0.474	325	1	0.991	0.00525	0.981	1.000
0.824	321	1	0.988	0.00607	0.976	1.000
.	.	.	.	.	.	.
12.936	41	1	0.217	0.02604	0.171	0.274
13.361	22	1	0.207	0.02665	0.161	0.266
13.936	1	1	0.000	NaN	NA	NA

If we only want the value of the Kaplan-Meier at specific time points, say at 5 and 10 years, we specify the `times` argument in the `summary.survfit` function

---

[20]Throughout we make use of R's object orientation when providing the actual code. Hence, we write `survfit` instead of `survfit.formula` etcetera.

```
summary(KM.curve, times=c(5,10))
```

with the result

time	n.risk	n.event	survival	std.err	lower95%CI	upper95%CI
5	215	89	0.713	0.0258	0.664	0.765
10	81	105	0.330	0.0284	0.279	0.391

Note that the value in `n.event` has changed into the total number of events until that time point.

The scale at which the confidence intervals are computed is chosen via the argument `conf.type` in the `survfit.formula` function. The default is `conf.type="log"`, which chooses the cumulative hazard scale as in (1.20). The log-log scale (1.21) and linear scale (1.18) can be chosen by specifying `"log-log"` and `"plain"` respectively.

The `plot.survfit` function makes a plot of the Kaplan-Meier. By default, the estimate is plotted on the scale of the survival curve $\widehat{\overline{F}}$, but specifying the argument `fun="event"` plots $\widehat{F}$ and `fun="cumhaz"` plots $\widehat{H}$. Figure 1.22 is obtained via

```
par(las=1) # this plots all axis labels horizontally
plot(KM.curve, fun="event", mark.time=FALSE, conf.int=FALSE,
                    xlab="time since HIV infection (years)",
                    ylab="overall cumulative incidence")
```

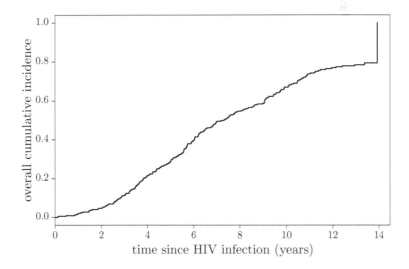

FIGURE 1.22
Estimate of cumulative incidence function for combined end point "AIDS/SI".

Without specifying `mark.time=FALSE`, "+" symbols are plotted at all the censoring times. The curve jumps to the value 1 at the end because the last event occurred when there were no further individuals at risk. The `plot.survfit` function does not stop automatically when there are only few individuals left in the risk set. If we do not want to show the last part of the curve, we can use the `xlim` argument, e.g. `xlim=c(0,12)`.

For a short summary of the fitted Cox model we use `print.coxph` via

```
fit.Cox
```

and obtain

```
Call:
coxph(formula = Surv(time, status != 0) ~ ccr5, data = aidssi)

          coef exp(coef) se(coef)      z       p
ccr5WM -0.701     0.496    0.186  -3.77 0.00016

Likelihood ratio test=16.5  on 1 df, p=4.95e-05  n= 324,
                     number of events= 220
   (5 observations deleted due to missingness)
```

For a detailed summary we write

```
summary(fit.Cox)
```

and obtain

```
Call:
coxph(formula = Surv(time, status != 0) ~ ccr5, data = aidssi)

  n= 324, number of events= 220
   (5 observations deleted due to missingness)

          coef exp(coef) se(coef)       z Pr(>|z|)
ccr5WM -0.7013    0.4959   0.1860  -3.771 0.000163 ***
---
Signif. codes:  0 "***" 0.001 "**" 0.01 "*" 0.05 "." 0.1 " " 1

          exp(coef) exp(-coef) lower .95 upper .95
ccr5WM       0.4959      2.016    0.3444     0.714

Concordance= 0.555  (se = 0.015 )
Rsquare= 0.05   (max possible= 0.999 )
Likelihood ratio test= 16.47  on 1 df,   p=4.953e-05
Wald test            = 14.22  on 1 df,   p=0.0001626
Score (logrank) test = 14.79  on 1 df,   p=0.0001204
```

We observe that, relative to the reference category WW, individuals with the CCR5-Δ32 deletion have a much slower progression to the combined event

AIDS/SI. We want to disentangle this effect with respect to both end points, which will be done via a competing risks analysis in later chapters.

We can test for proportionality via scaled Schoenfeld residuals by using the `cox.zph` function:

```
cox.zph(fit.Cox)
```

gives

```
        rho  chisq    p
ccr5WM 0.0291 0.183 0.669
```

and we conclude that there is no indication of non-proportionality.

For prediction based on the results from a Cox model we use the `survfit.coxph` function. By default, it chooses the reference values for the co-variables (see Page 39). If we want to choose a specific combination of values, we create a data frame with these combinations.

```
new.indiv <- data.frame(ccr5=c("WW","WM"))
```

We summarize the estimated survival curves via the `summary.survfit` function. We have to select the curve for each value separately using square brackets via

```
summary(survfit(fit.Cox, newdata=new.indiv)[1], times=c(5,10))
summary(survfit(fit.Cox, newdata=new.indiv)[2], times=c(5,10))
```

For the first group, the reference value `WW`, we obtain

time	n.risk	n.event	survival	std.err	lower 95% CI	upper 95% CI
5	214	88	0.686	0.0283	0.633	0.744
10	81	104	0.279	0.0301	0.226	0.345

We see that the `WM` value gives a higher survival curve:

time	n.risk	n.event	survival	std.err	lower 95% CI	upper 95% CI
5	214	88	0.830	0.0304	0.772	0.891
10	81	104	0.531	0.0587	0.428	0.659

Plotting the survival curve can be done for both values at once:

```
plot(survfit(fit.Cox, newdata=new.indiv))
```

1.11.5 Log-rank test

The log-rank test is performed with the `survdiff` function.

```
survdiff(Surv(time,status!=0)~ccr5, data=aidssi)
```

We can choose other weight functions of the form $\widehat{F}^{\rho}$ via the `rho` argument, the log-rank test has the default $\rho = 0$. The output compares observed and expected number of events as in (1.24):

```
n=324, 5 observations deleted due to missingness.

          N Observed Expected (O-E)^2/E (O-E)^2/V
ccr5=WW 259      185    159.9      3.93      14.8
ccr5=WM  65       35     60.1     10.47      14.8


 Chisq= 14.8  on 1 degrees of freedom, p= 0.00012
```

In correspondence with the Cox model, we observe that individuals with the CCR5-Δ32 deletion have significantly fewer events than expected under the null hypothesis that both groups have the same time-to-event distribution.

In the current version of the survival package, the `survdiff` function does not allow the event time data to be in counting process format. If we want to perform the log-rank test for data that have the counting process format, we can use the score test based on a Cox model. See the example on Page 101.

When testing whether the curves are different, it is recommended to calculate and plot the survival curves as well. We obtain one Kaplan-Meier curve per value of CCR5 via

```
KM.ccr5 <- survfit(Surv(time,status!=0)~ccr5, data=aidssi)
```

We select both curves in `summary.survfit` and `plot.survfit` via square brackets. The summary of the estimate for the `WW` value is obtained via

```
summary(KM.ccr5[1])
```

1.12   Computer practicals

The data we use comes from the EBMT registry and contains information on 1977 patients who received an allogeneic bone marrow transplantation. We refer to Section 1.2.3 for some background information. Time is measured in days from transplantation. The EBMT risk score is called **score**. The data can be found in the `mstate` package. Make sure that you have installed `mstate`. We load the package and the data via

```
library(mstate)
data(ebmt1)
```

1. **A first look at the data** Have a look at the help file of the `ebmt1` data set to get information on the meaning of the variables and their possible values.

    Inspect the data by looking at the first couple of individuals or by viewing the complete data set. How many rows and columns does the data set have? Look at the type of the variables (count, continuous or categorical).

Summarize all the variables. Why are there 1521 NA's in the variable **yrel**? How many relapses were observed and how many deaths?

2. **Some data preparation** In the `ebmt1` data set, information with respect to relapse and death is given in separate columns. In a competing risks analysis, the usual data presentation is via a single time and status column.

Add two more columns to the `ebmt1` data set. One column, to be called **time**, contains the time of the first of the two events, relapse and death, or the time of censoring if neither was observed. Use year instead of day as time unit. The second column, to be called **stat**, is a column that has the value 0 for right censored individuals, 1 if there was a relapse and 2 if the individual died without having had a relapse. You can add a third column that explains the meaning of 0, 1 and 2.

R Hint. The function `pmin` computes the minimum value of two of more columns of numeric variables. It is a vectorized function, meaning that the minimum per row is computed. Since death never occurs before relapse, we can see which individuals are censored via the **srvstat** column. There are many ways to add the columns, but one efficient way is the following.

```
ebmt1 <- within(ebmt1,{
  time <-  pmin(srv,rel)/365.25
  stat <-   ifelse(rel<srv,relstat,srvstat*2)
  type <- factor(stat,
                  labels=c("Event-free","Relapse","Death"))
})
```

3. **Estimation of overall cumulative incidence** Compute the Kaplan-Meier estimator for relapse-free survival. Relapse-free survival means that the individual neither had a relapse nor died, i.e. both end points are combined as an event. Obtain the estimates of relapse-free survival at one and five years. Plot the estimate of the cumulative incidence (the complement of the Kaplan-Meier survival curve).

4. **A Cox model for relapse-free survival** Fit a Cox model for the effect of the EBMT score on relapse-free survival. Locate the hazard ratios. What is your conclusion with respect to the effect of the EBMT score?

Test whether the effect of the EBMT score is non-proportional.

5. **Log-rank test** Use the log-rank test to investigate whether the EBMT score influences relapse-free survival. Make a plot of the cumulative hazard per level of the EBMT score.

2

Competing Risks; Nonparametric Estimation

2.1 Introduction

A typical survival analysis in medical research has two components. First, the Kaplan-Meier is calculated as a nonparametric estimate of the time-to-event distribution for the total population that the sample represents. If there are a few subgroups of main interest, such as a treatment and placebo group in a clinical trial, it is calculated separately for each of them. In order to know whether the subgroups have a different time-to-event distribution, a log-rank test is performed. Next, the effect of covariables is quantified via a regression model; the Cox proportional hazards model is the most commonly used one.

The same components can be distinguished in competing risks and multi-state settings. This chapter explains nonparametric estimation of the cause-specific cumulative incidence, and it describes two log-rank tests. Chapter 3 covers nonparametric estimation in the multi-state setting.

If there is left truncation and/or right censoring, estimation is usually based on the hazard. In competing risks settings, two hazards can be defined, the cause-specific hazard and the subdistribution hazard. They are defined formally in Section 2.2. We show how they relate to the cause-specific cumulative incidence function F_k. In Sections 2.3 and 2.4 we explain the nonparametric estimation of both hazards. We introduce three estimators of F_k. Although they look different, algebraically they are the same: they give exactly the same result. The classical one is based on the estimator of the cause-specific hazard (Section 2.3). It is a special case of the Aalen-Johansen estimator of the transition probability in multi-state models (Chapter 3). A second form is based on an estimator of the subdistribution hazard (2.17). This form is attractive because it has the same product-limit structure as the classical Kaplan-Meier, which allows us to use standard software. The third one is not based on hazards but calculates the cumulative frequency of observed events (2.19). As a special case we address estimation with completely observed data, i.e. when there is neither censoring nor left truncation (Section 2.4.1). Although this situation is uncommon, it is explained because it shows the basic structure of both the product-limit form and the cumulative frequency form. In the more general case, the only thing that changes is the inclusion of weights that correct for the missing information due to left truncation and/or right censoring. If you are not interested in the calculation and interpretation of the weights, you can skip Section 2.4 from 2.4.2 onwards. In Section 2.5 we describe how to obtain confidence intervals and in Section 2.6 we introduce the competing risks analogues of the log-rank test, one for each type of hazard.

We refer to Section 1.7 for all the notation that is used. Unless specified otherwise, we assume that the entry and censoring times (V_i, C_i) are independent of both the event time and the event type (T_i, E_i).

2.2 Theoretical relations

There are two ways to write the cause-specific cumulative incidence via hazards. One interprets the competing risks situation as a multi-state model and combines the cause-specific hazards of all competing risks. We write (T, E) to represent the event time and event type. The other ignores the competing events and only considers the distribution of time to the event of interest. Since the cumulative probability does not go up to one, it is called a subdistribution. We write T_k for the time to the event of interest $E = k$.

Just as in classical survival analysis (Section 1.8), definitions and relations differ slightly between continuous and discrete distributions. Since the number of observed events is finite, nonparametric estimation is based on the discrete situation.

2.2.1 The multi-state approach; cause-specific hazards

The cause-specific hazard quantifies the progression rate to a specific end point for those that are at risk. If T has a continuous distribution it is defined as

$$\lambda_k(t) = \lim_{\Delta t \downarrow 0} \frac{P(t \le T < t + \Delta t, E = k \mid T \ge t)}{\Delta t}, \tag{2.1}$$

while the definition for discrete T is

$$\lambda_k(t_l) = P(T = t_l, E = k \mid T \ge t_l). \tag{2.2}$$

If we add all cause-specific hazards we obtain the overall hazard (e.g. the sum of the cause-specific mortality rates is the overall mortality rate). We show it formally for the continuous case:

$$\sum_{e=1}^{K} \lambda_e(t) = \lim_{\Delta t \downarrow 0} \frac{\sum_{e=1}^{K} P(t \le T < t + \Delta t, E = e \mid T \ge t)}{\Delta t}$$

$$= \lim_{\Delta t \downarrow 0} \frac{P(t \le T < t + \Delta t \mid T \ge t)}{\Delta t} = h(t). \tag{2.3}$$

Similar to (1.4) and (1.8), we define the integrated/cumulative cause-specific hazard as $\Lambda_k(t) = \int_0^t \lambda_k(s)ds$ for continuous distributions and $\Lambda_k(t) = \sum_{t_i \le t} \lambda_k(t_i)$ for discrete distributions.

The cause-specific cumulative incidence is determined by all cause-specific hazards. For continuous distributions we have

$$F_k(t) = \mathrm{P}(T \leq t, E = k) = \int_0^t \overline{F}(s)\lambda_k(s)ds \qquad (2.4)$$

and for discrete distributions the relation is

$$F_k(t) = \mathrm{P}(T \leq t, E = k) = \sum_{t_l \leq t} \overline{F}(t_l-)\lambda_k(t_l). \qquad (2.5)$$

These relations can be seen to hold as follows. The probability that an event of type k occurs at some time s is a product of two terms (Figure 2.1). One is the probability that no event happened before time s, i.e. $\mathrm{P}(T \geq s)$, and the other is the probability of the event of type k to occur at time s given that the event has not happened yet, which is the cause-specific hazard $\lambda_k(s)$.

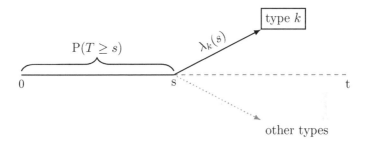

FIGURE 2.1
The probability to progress to event k at time s is a product of the probabilities $\mathrm{P}(T \geq s)$ and $\lambda_k(s)$.

The probability to remain free of any event until just before time s is the overall survival function, $\mathrm{P}(T \geq s) = \overline{F}(s-)$. For a continuous distribution the survival function does not have jumps and we have $\overline{F}(s-) = \overline{F}(s)$. Relations (2.4) and (2.5) are obtained by combining all possible time points between 0 and t.

If we add all cause-specific cumulative incidences we obtain the overall cumulative incidence (e.g. the sum of the death specific cumulative probabilities is the overall death risk). In formula form:

$$\sum_{e=1}^K F_e(t) = \sum_{e=1}^K \mathrm{P}(T \leq t, E = e) = \mathrm{P}(T \leq t) = F(t). \qquad (2.6)$$

The overall survival function relates to the cause-specific hazards via

$$\overline{F}(t) = \exp\left\{-\int_0^t h(s)ds\right\} = \exp\left\{-\sum_{e=1}^K \int_0^t \lambda_e(s)ds\right\}$$

$$= \prod_{e=1}^K \exp\left\{-\int_0^t \lambda_e(s)ds\right\}. \tag{2.7}$$

In this expression we see reflected what was explained before: the cause-specific hazards can be interpreted as marginal hazards if and only if they are independent. If the competing risks are not independent, then the product property (2.7) still holds, but it no longer specifies an independence property; the hazards are cause-specific and $\exp\{-\Lambda_e(t)\}$ does not specify a survival function as in (1.9).

Since the cause-specific cumulative incidence for one event type k is determined by all cause-specific hazards, there is no one-to-one correspondence between the cause-specific hazard and the cause-specific cumulative incidence for the same cause. As a consequence, it can happen that the cause-specific hazard is lower for a subgroup over the whole time range, whereas the cause-specific cumulative incidence is higher for at least part of the time scale. In Section 5.2 we will see an example.

2.2.2   The subdistribution approach

The hazard that does have a one-to-one relation with the cause-specific cumulative incidence is the subdistribution hazard. For continuous distributions the subdistribution hazard $h_k(t)$ for type k is defined as

$$h_k(t) = \lim_{\Delta t \downarrow 0} \frac{\mathrm{P}(t \le T_k < t + \Delta t \,|\, T_k \ge t)}{\Delta t}, \tag{2.8}$$

and for discrete distributions we define

$$h_k(t_l) = \mathrm{P}(T_k = t_l \,|\, T_k \ge t_l). \tag{2.9}$$

The integrated/cumulative subdistribution hazard is defined as $H_k(t) = \int_0^t h_k(s)ds$ and $H_k(t) = \sum_{t_i \le t} h_k(t_i)$ for continuous and discrete distributions respectively.

The relation between subdistribution hazard and cumulative incidence F_k can be expressed for continuous distributions as

$$\overline{F_k}(t) = \exp\left\{-\int_0^t h_k(s)ds\right\}$$

and for discrete distributions as

$$\overline{F_k}(t) = \prod_{t_l \le t}\left\{1 - h_k(t_l)\right\}. \tag{2.10}$$

These relations are the same as (1.9) and (1.5) for the classical survival setting.

We rewrite the subdistribution hazard in terms of the multi-state variable (T, E). For discrete distributions we obtain

$$
\begin{aligned}
h_k(t_l) = \mathrm{P}(T_k = t_l \mid T_k \geq t_l) &= \frac{\mathrm{P}(T_k = t_l)}{\mathrm{P}(T_k \geq t_l)} \\
&= \frac{\mathrm{P}(T = t_l, E = k)}{\mathrm{P}\{T \geq t_l \text{ or } (T < t_l, E \neq k)\}} \\
&= \frac{\mathrm{P}(T = t_l, E = k)}{\overline{F}(t_l-) + \sum_{l \neq k} F_l(t_l-)} .
\end{aligned}
\tag{2.11}
$$

We see what is different from the cause-specific hazard: the term in the denominator not only contains the probability to be event-free just before t_l, but also the probability to have experienced a competing event at an earlier time point.

Subdistribution hazard and cause-specific hazard are related via

$$
\lambda_k(t) \times \overline{F}(t-) = h_k(t) \times \overline{F_k}(t-) .
\tag{2.12}
$$

This result not only holds for the theoretical distributions [13] but also for the nonparametric estimators [37], which can be interpreted as empirical discrete distributions.

2.3   Estimation based on cause-specific hazard

The cause-specific hazard quantifies the progression rate to the end point of interest in a setting in which individuals can also progress to one of the competing end points. If an individual experiences a competing event, he is no longer at risk for experiencing the event of interest and he leaves the risk set. Therefore, the cause-specific hazard λ_k is estimated by counting the number of events of the type of interest, divided by the observed number at risk:

$$
\widehat{\lambda_k}(t_{(i)}) = \frac{d_k(t_{(i)})}{r(t_{(i)})} .
\tag{2.13}
$$

If we can assume that the occurrence of the competing events is noninformative for the event of interest, the marginal hazard is estimated in the same way. However, if the occurrence of another event is informative, we no longer estimate the marginal hazard but only the cause-specific hazard. Interpreted as an estimate of the cause-specific hazard, we do not assume that individuals who experience a competing event can be represented by the individuals that

remain in follow-up. For example, cardiovascular disease (cvd) and chronic renal failure are serious long-term complications of diabetes, and both can cause
mortality. We can estimate cvd-specific mortality rates in diabetes patients,
even though diabetes patients that die of cvd are also more prone to die of
renal failure. This estimate of cvd-specific mortality does not quantify the
cvd-specific mortality in the hypothetical situation in which diabetes patients
cannot die of renal failure.

The cumulative cause-specific hazard until time t is estimated by the sum
of the cause-specific hazard estimates until time t: $\widehat{\Lambda}_k(t) = \sum_{t_{(i)} \leq t} \widehat{\lambda}_k(t_{(i)})$. It
is called the Nelson-Aalen estimator.

The estimator of the cause-specific cumulative incidence function is based
on relation (2.5) between cause-specific hazard and cause-specific cumulative
incidence:

$$\widehat{F}_k^{\text{AJ}}(t) = \sum_{t_{(i)} \leq t} \widehat{\overline{F}}^{\text{PL}}(t_{(i)}-) \times \widehat{\lambda}_k(t_{(i)}). \tag{2.14}$$

$\widehat{\overline{F}}^{\text{PL}}(t_{(i)}-)$ is the Kaplan-Meier estimate of the overall cumulative incidence
that combines all event types:

$$\widehat{\overline{F}}^{\text{PL}}(t_{(i)}-) = \prod_{t_{(j)} < t_{(i)}} \left\{ 1 - \frac{d(t_{(j)})}{r(t_{(j)})} \right\}.$$

(2.14) is a special case of the Aalen-Johansen estimator (3.9) of the transition
probability in a multi-state model. Therefore we use the superscript AJ.

What holds for the theoretical distributions also holds for the estimators:
the estimate of the overall cumulative incidence is equal to the sum of all cause-
specific cumulative incidence estimates. This can also be shown by looking at
the jump sizes. Since (2.14) is a sum of terms, its jump at $t_{(i)}$ is equal to

$$\widehat{F}_k^{\text{AJ}}(t_{(i)}) - \widehat{F}_k^{\text{AJ}}(t_{(i)}-) = \widehat{\overline{F}}^{\text{PL}}(t_{(i)}-) \times \frac{d_k(t_{(i)})}{r(t_{(i)})}. \tag{2.15}$$

Combining the jump sizes over all event types, we obtain:

$$\sum_{e=1}^{K} [\widehat{F}_e^{\text{AJ}}(t_{(i)}) - \widehat{F}_e^{\text{AJ}}(t_{(i)}-)] = \widehat{\overline{F}}^{\text{PL}}(t_{(i)}-) \times \frac{\sum_{e=1}^{K} d_e(t_{(i)})}{r(t_{(i)})}$$

$$= \widehat{\overline{F}}^{\text{PL}}(t_{(i)}-) \times \frac{d(t_{(i)})}{r(t_{(i)})}$$

This is equal to the jump size in the Kaplan-Meier estimate of the overall
survival function, which follows from (1.3).

An example

Detailed explanations by example of how (2.14) is calculated can be found in
several papers (e.g. [53, 87]). We give another example, which is also used in
Section 2.4 as an example of the calculations with the other two forms.

Suppose the following data:

- There are 200 individuals, and two competing causes of death A and B. Our interest is in cause A.

  - 115 individuals die of A (60 at 2 years, 55 at 6 years)
  - 85 individuals die of B (40 at 4 years, 45 at 8 years)

  With complete data, we can use the frequency estimator that is explained in Section 2.4.1 and obtain $\widehat{F_A}^{\text{EC}}(2) = \frac{60}{200}$ and $\widehat{F_A}^{\text{EC}}(6) = \frac{115}{200}$.

- The observed data is incomplete

  - 50 individuals are censored after 5 years
  - 100 individuals enter 3 years after the time origin (if they are still event free)

The complete information, including the late entry and right censoring, is shown in Figure 2.2. Events are denoted by circles. Events that end in an open circle are not observed, due to right censoring at the start of the dashed lines. The unobserved period before late entry is denoted by a dotted line and the time of entry by "(". The 25 individuals in the first row, who would enter at 3 years, are not observed at all since they had event A before they entered the study. Hence the late entry leads to left truncation. In Figure 2.3 we show the observed data.

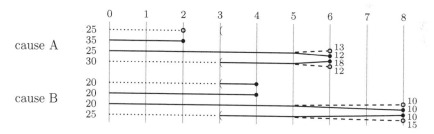

FIGURE 2.2
Example of calculations with competing risks: graphical representation of the complete information. Information that is not observed is shown via dotted lines (late entry) and dashed lines (right censoring).

In Table 2.1, we calculate the Aalen-Johansen estimate of the cause-specific cumulative incidence for cause A. The estimate $\widehat{\lambda}_A$ of the cause-specific hazard for cause A has a value unequal to zero at $t = 2$ and $t = 6$ only. The estimate of the overall hazard $\widehat{h}$ additionally has a value unequal to zero at $t = 4$, when the competing event occurs. Next, we calculate the Kaplan-Meier $\widehat{F}^{\text{PL}}$ for both end points combined. In the last line we use (2.14). Note that $\widehat{P}(T \geq t) = \widehat{F}^{\text{PL}}(t-)$ is determined by the event times before t.

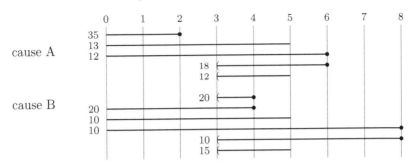

FIGURE 2.3
Example of calculations with competing risks: graphical representation of the observed data. Lines not ending with a closed circle correspond to right censored observations.

TABLE 2.1
Detailed calculation of $\widehat{F_A}^{AJ}(2)$ and $\widehat{F_A}^{AJ}(6)$

	2 years	**4 years**	**6 years**
$\widehat{\lambda_A}(t)$	$\frac{35}{100}$	0	$\frac{30}{50}$
$\widehat{h}(t)$	$\frac{35}{100}$	$\frac{40}{140}$	$\frac{30}{50}$
$\widehat{P}(T \geq t)$	1	$\left(1 - \frac{35}{100}\right) = \frac{65}{100}$ $\frac{65}{100} \times \left(1 - \frac{40}{140}\right) = \frac{65}{140}$
$\widehat{F_A}^{AJ}(t)$	$1 \times \frac{35}{100} = \frac{35}{100}$	$\frac{35}{100} + \frac{65}{100} \times 0 = \frac{35}{100}$	$\frac{35}{100} + \frac{65}{140} \times \frac{30}{50} = \frac{22}{35}$

Display formats

As an example, we show the estimates of the cause-specific cumulative incidence of AIDS and SI as first events, based on the `aidssi` data set (see Section 1.11.1). When showing the results graphically, there are several options.

In Figure 2.4 we use the *alternate* display format. One outcome, SI, is plotted as the "survival" curve $\overline{F}_{SI}$, starting at one and decreasing, and the other one, AIDS, as the cumulative incidence curve F_{AIDS}, starting at zero and going up. This format can be informative if there are two event types.

In the figure we also show the "marginal" Kaplan-Meier curves that are based on the estimate of the "marginal" hazard[1]. These curves are steeper than the cause-specific curves. We also see that the curves cross, which can never happen with cause-specific cumulative incidence curves; they always add up to a number ≤ 1.

Another option is the *stacked* format. In Figure 2.5, the AIDS-specific curve F_{AIDS} is the same as in Figure 2.4. The SI-specific curve is plotted on

---

[1]We write marginal in quotes because it probably does not estimate the marginal distribution, due to informative censoring.

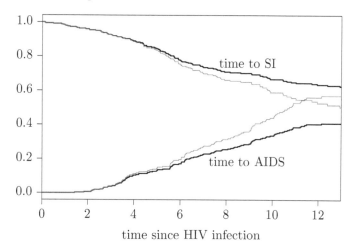

FIGURE 2.4

Estimated cause-specific cumulative incidence function for AIDS and SI as first events, alternate display format (solid black lines). The "marginal" Kaplan-Meier curves are shown in gray.

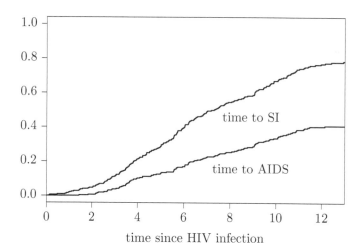

FIGURE 2.5

Estimate of cause-specific cumulative incidence for AIDS and SI as first events, in a stacked display format.

top of it. The difference between both curves quantifies the probability to have progressed to SI. Using (2.6) we derive that the upper curve is equal to the overall cumulative incidence: $F_{AIDS} + F_{SI} = F$. Therefore the upper curve can be obtained by calculating the overall Kaplan-Meier in which both end points are combined. This format is informative if we want to emphasize how all event types add up to the overall risk. It can be used with any number of competing event types.

In the *overlaid* format we plot the estimates for the different end points in the same manner. This format is informative when comparing the progression to the different competing risks. An example is Figure 2.12 from Exercise 8 (Page 89), in which risk of symptomatic cardiac events and death from other causes are plotted. A fourth option is to plot the cumulative incidence for each end point in a separate figure or panel. This *separate* format is useful if we are interested in the difference by subgroup for each end point separately. An example is Figure 4.4 on Page 169, in which the main interest is in the relation between HCV status and the progression for each cause of death separately.

2.4   Estimation: the subdistribution approach

The Aalen-Johansen estimator is the classical approach to nonparametric estimation of the cause-specific cumulative incidence. We describe two alternatives that are based on the subdistribution.

One uses the product-limit Formula (2.10), which is based on the subdistribution hazard. The estimator of the subdistribution hazard is motivated by expression (2.11). Contrary to the cause-specific hazard, individuals that experienced an earlier competing event remain included in the denominator. For estimation this entails that the occurrence of a competing event is ignored and such individuals remain in the risk set until the time at which they would have been censored for another reason than the competing event. This suggests the following estimator

$$\widehat{h_k}(t_{(i)}) = \frac{d_k(t_{(i)})}{r^*(t_{(i)})}, \tag{2.16}$$

with $r^*(t_{(i)})$ the extended number at risk. The estimator of the cause-specific cumulative incidence becomes

$$\widehat{F}_k^{PL}(t) = \prod_{t_{(j)} \leq t} \left\{ 1 - \frac{d_k(t_{(j)})}{r^*(t_{(j)})} \right\}. \tag{2.17}$$

Since it has a product-limit form, we use the superscript PL. Note that $r^*(t_{(j)})$ is never smaller than $r(t_{(j)})$, and therefore the classical Kaplan-Meier is always at least as steep as the estimator of the cause-specific cumulative incidence.

Unless all censoring is administrative, we don't know the censoring time. We use the observed censoring pattern to estimate the distribution of censoring times. Based on this estimate, we can perform multiple imputation of censoring times [86]. We describe an alternative approach in which an individual that experiences a competing event remains in the risk set with a weight that changes over time according to the estimated probability of remaining uncensored.

We also need to correct for left truncation. Since the occurrence of a competing event does not remove an individual from the risk set, an individual that experienced a competing event before he became at risk needs to be included in the denominator from his entry time onwards. Typically, this individual is not observed and the time he would have entered is unknown. We use weights such that individuals that are not missed and experience a competing event represent individuals that are missed due to the occurrence of a competing event before entry.

We first define the general structure of the weight functions. Let $\widehat{\Gamma}$ and $\widehat{\Phi}$ denote estimators of the censoring and entry time distributions. The contribution $\omega_l(t_{(i)})$ of individual l to the risk set $r^*(t_{(i)})$ is equal to

$$\omega_l(t_{(i)}) = \begin{cases} 1 & \text{if event-free and under observation until } t_{(i)} \\ \dfrac{\widehat{\Gamma}(t_{(i)}-)}{\widehat{\Gamma}(t_{(j)}-)} \dfrac{\widehat{\Phi}(t_{(i)}-)}{\widehat{\Phi}(t_{(j)}-)} & \text{if competing event observed at } t_{(j)} < t_{(i)} \\ 0 & \text{otherwise} \end{cases}$$

(2.18)

In Section 2.4.3.2 we give a more formal derivation of this weight function and in Section 2.4.4 we make some remarks on the interpretation.

A third approach is to estimate the cause-specific cumulative incidence directly as a cumulative frequency of observed events, without using hazards. With right censored and left truncated data we use the same estimates $\widehat{\Gamma}$ and $\widehat{\Phi}$ to define a weighted form as

$$\widehat{F}_k^{\text{EC}}(t) = \frac{1}{\widehat{N}} \sum_{t_{(j)} \le t} \frac{d_k(t_{(j)})}{\widehat{\Gamma}(t_{(j)}-) \times \widehat{\Phi}(t_{(j)}-)}, \tag{2.19}$$

with constant $\widehat{N}$ defined as

$$\widehat{N} = \sum_{i=1}^{n} \frac{d(t_{(i)})}{\widehat{\Phi}(t_{(i)}-)} + \sum_{j=1}^{m} \frac{m_j}{\widehat{\Phi}(c_{(j)}-)}. \tag{2.20}$$

m_j is the number of censorings at $c_{(j)}$, see Section 1.7. Since it is similar in structure to the empirical cumulative distribution function (ECDF) in (1.14), we use the superscript EC. The first term in $\widehat{N}$ is a sum over all individuals who had their event observed (of any type), the second term is a sum over all individuals that were censored. Both are weighted to correct for left truncation. $\widehat{N}$ is equal to N in the absence of left truncation. If everybody enters at the time origin, $\Phi(t)$ is equal to one everywhere, and because every individual is either censored or has an event, we obtain $\widehat{N} = \sum_{i=1}^{n} d(t_{(i)}) + \sum_{j=1}^{m} m_j = N$. With left truncated data, $\widehat{N}$ is larger than N and can be interpreted as an estimate of the total sample size, including the individuals that are missed due to left truncation (see Section 2.4.4).

In Section 2.4.2 we define $\widehat{T}$ and $\widehat{\Phi}$ in such a way that both the PL form in (2.17) and the ECDF form in (2.19) become algebraically equivalent to the Aalen-Johansen estimator:

$$\widehat{F_k}^{\text{AJ}}(t) = \widehat{F_k}^{\text{EC}}(t) = \widehat{F_k}^{\text{PL}}(t) \qquad \text{for all time points } t. \qquad (2.21)$$

2.4.1   Estimation with complete follow-up

We first describe the ECDF and PL forms for the situation with a complete follow-up, in which both have a very simple structure. Follow-up is complete until time t if there is no left truncation and if all censoring occurs after t, i.e. every individual is either still at risk or the event, of whatever type, has been observed. Then we know that all individuals that had a competing event would still be at risk at time t if the event had not happened.

As an example, consider the (artificial) data set in Table 2.2 of 146 patients with complete information on infection during their hospital stay and discharge for the first seven weeks.

TABLE 2.2
Competing risks data with complete follow-up during the first seven weeks

	week	0-1	1-2	2-3	3-4	4-5	5-6	6-7	> 7
infection:	number	1	2	6	11	9	11	2	18
	cumulative	1	3	9	20	29	40	42	60
discharge:	number	5	9	6	6	9	12	4	35
	cumulative	5	14	20	26	35	47	51	86

The probability of becoming infected in the hospital within six weeks is simply estimated as the cumulative frequency of observed infection events,

$$\widehat{P}(\text{infection} \leq 6 \text{ weeks}) = 40/146,$$

and similarly for discharge without infection,

$$\widehat{P}(\text{discharge} \leq 6 \text{ weeks}) = 47/146.$$

Note that individuals that are observed to experience the competing event remain in the denominator. The general formula for the ECDF form with completely observed data is

$$\widehat{F_k}^{\text{EC}}(t) = \frac{\sum_{t_{(j)} \leq t} d_k(t_{(j)})}{N}. \qquad (2.22)$$

This formula is similar to (1.14) for the setting with one event type. It is easy to show that this ECDF form is equivalent to the Aalen-Johansen estimator (Exercise 6 in Section 2.8).

When using the PL form based on an estimator of the subdistribution hazard, the same principle applies. Only individuals that experience the event of interest are removed from the risk set. Therefore, the extended number at risk $r^*(t_{(i)})$ is equal to the number of individuals that did not yet experience the event of interest, i.e. are still at risk or had a competing event before $t_{(i)}$. Using a similar argument as on Page 33 for the Kaplan-Meier, the PL form can be shown to be equivalent to $\widehat{F}_k^{\mathrm{EC}}$.

Complete data over the whole follow-up time is not very common. We may encounter it in situations in which the time scale of the processes is short. An example is death and discharge as competing events in an intensive care unit [29]. Another reason to consider complete data is because results are easier to interpret, while the basic structure of the estimators does not change compared to data with left truncation and right censoring[2].

2.4.2 A special choice for $\widehat{\Gamma}$ and $\widehat{\Phi}$

We define the $\widehat{\Gamma}$ and $\widehat{\Phi}$ that make the ECDF and PL forms algebraically equivalent to the Aalen-Johansen estimator.

Right censored data.

The $\widehat{\Gamma}$ that corrects for right censoring has a product-limit form that reverses the role of events and censorings:

$$\widehat{\Gamma}(t) = \prod_{j:c_{(j)} \leq t} \left\{ 1 - \frac{m_j}{r(c_{(j)})} \right\}. \tag{2.23}$$

If there is no left truncation, or if right censoring and left truncation are independent, it can be seen as an estimator of $\overline{\Gamma}(t)$, the probability to remain free of censoring until time t (see the discussion in Section 2.4.4 on Page 76).

In Figure 2.6, we show the information in the example data set when the role of event and censoring is reversed compared to Figure 2.3: the lines representing censored individuals end with a closed circle and the lines representing events don't. The only censoring, which is treated as event, occurs at $c = 5$. The estimate of the censoring hazard at that time is

$$\frac{13 + 12 + 10 + 15}{13 + 12 + 18 + 12 + 10 + 10 + 10 + 15} = \frac{50}{100} = 0.5 \,.$$

Hence we have $\widehat{\Gamma}^{\mathrm{PL}}(t) = 1$ for $t < 5$ and $\widehat{\Gamma}^{\mathrm{PL}}(t) = 1 - 0.5 = 0.5$ thereafter.

---

[2] In statistics, the parameters that describe the censoring and truncation process are called nuisance parameters.

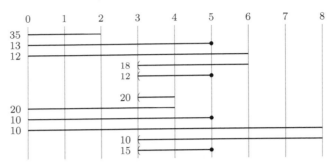

FIGURE 2.6
Example of calculations with competing risks: graphical representation of the
data in which censorings are treated as events and events as censorings.

Left truncated data.

The $\widehat{\varPhi}$ that corrects for left truncation has a product-limit form that reverses
the role of events/censorings and late entries:

$$\widehat{\varPhi}(t) = \prod_{v_{(j)} > t} \left\{ 1 - \frac{w_j}{r(v_{(j)})} \right\}. \tag{2.24}$$

w_j is the number of entries at $v_{(j)}$ (see Section 1.7). The structure of the
formula is slightly different from the regular product-limit form: the value at
time t is a product over entry times that are *larger* than t.

If there are no right censored data, or if entry time V and censoring time
C are independent, it estimates the entry time distribution $\varPhi(t) = \mathrm{P}(V \leq
t)$. $X_i = \min(T_i, C_i)$ induces right truncation of the entry times: entries are
observed if $V_i < X_i$. While left truncation causes small event times to be
underrepresented (see Section 1.3.3), right truncation causes large event times
to be underrepresented: small event times V_i are more likely than large event
times to be smaller than X_i, hence to be observed. Right truncated event
time data can be analysed by reversing the time scale: $-V_i$ is observed if
$-X_i < -V_i$. Now we are back in the situation of left truncated data: "event
times" $-V_i$ are observed if $-X_i \leq -V_i$. All values are below zero, but that
is not an essential restriction. And such data can always be made to have
positive values by adding a number that is larger than all observed values X_i.
Hence, the distribution $\varPhi$ of V is estimated via

$$\widehat{\mathrm{P}}(V \leq t) = \widehat{\mathrm{P}}(-V \geq -t) = \prod_{j:-v_{(j)} < -t} \left\{ 1 - \frac{w_j}{r(v_{(j)})} \right\}$$

$$= \prod_{j:v_{(j)} > t} \left\{ 1 - \frac{w_j}{r(v_{(j)})} \right\}.$$

Since we estimate $\widehat{P}(V \leq t)$ instead of $\widehat{P}(V < t)$, the product is over all $v_{(j)}$ that are strictly larger than t.

The data needed for the calculation of $\widehat{\Phi}^{\text{PL}}$ in our example data set is shown in Figure 2.7. Right truncation as caused by the events and censorings is denoted by ")". The entries, which play the role of events, occur at $v = 0$ and $v = 3$.

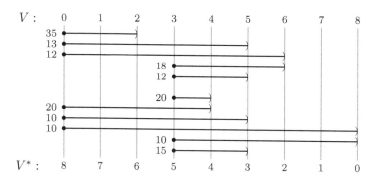

FIGURE 2.7
Example of calculations with competing risks: graphical representation of the data with entry treated as event and events and censorings inducing right truncation.

At $v = 3$ we have

$$\frac{w_2}{r(v_{(2)})} = \frac{18 + 12 + 20 + 10 + 15}{13 + 12 + 18 + 12 + 20 + 20 + 10 + 10 + 10 + 15} = \frac{75}{140},$$

hence $\widehat{\Phi}(t) = 1 - 75/140 = 65/140$ for $0 \leq t < 3$ and $\widehat{\Phi}(t) = 1$ thereafter. Hence, the probability to be observed from $t = 0$ onwards, $P(V \leq 0)$, is estimated to be $65/140$ and the estimate of the probability to enter at $t = 3$ is $75/140$. We may create the variable $V^* = -V + 8$, which transforms right truncated into left truncated event time data that don't have a negative value. Events or censorings occur at $v^* = 0, 2, 3, 4$ and 6. The only entries occur at $v^* = 5$ and $v^* = 8$. Hence $\widehat{P}(V^* > v^*) = 1$ for $v^* < 5$, $\widehat{P}(V^* > v^*) = \frac{65}{140}$ for $5 \leq v^* < 8$ and $\widehat{P}(V^* > v^*) = 0$ for $v^* \geq 8$, translating into $\widehat{P}(V < v) = 1$ for $v > 3$, $\widehat{P}(V < v) = \frac{65}{140}$ for $0 < v \leq 3$ and $\widehat{P}(V < v) = 0$ for $v \leq 0$.

2.4.3 The ECDF and PL forms

In this section, we calculate the ECDF and PL forms in our example data set, using the weights based on Section 2.4.2. And we give a more formal justification for the weights (2.18) in the estimator of the subdistribution hazard.

2.4.3.1   The ECDF form

The ECDF form was first introduced for the classical survival setting with right censored data only [88]. A similar form was derived if there is only left truncation [93]. Later, both forms were combined if right censoring and left truncation occur in the same data set and it was extended to the competing risks setting [37]. The ECDF form has not been used very often. We use the ECDF form when deriving our estimator of the subdistribution hazard in Section 2.4.3.2. From a practical perspective, the ECDF form can be attractive when the sole interest is in the cumulative scale. It circumvents the use of the hazard. The cause-specific hazard has the disadvantage that it does not directly translate to the cumulative scale. The subdistribution hazard has been criticized for not being a true rate and being hard to interpret (see Section 2.4.4). Also, the ECDF form provides the basis for an alternative to the log-rank test that is likely to have have more power with nonproportional hazards. And it provides the basis for estimation in the proportional odds model (Section 5.4).

We show the calculations for our example data set. Late entries only occur at $t = 3$. Hence $\widehat{\Phi}(t) = 1$ at the event times $t = 4$ (with 40 events of type B), $t = 6$ (30 events of type A) and $t = 8$ (20 events of type A), as well as at the censor time $t = 5$ (50 censorings). Only the individuals with an event at $t = 2$ (35 events of type A) are reweighted by $1/\widehat{\Phi}(2-) = 1/\widehat{\Phi}(2) = 140/65$. Hence we obtain $\widehat{N} = 35 \times 140/65 + 140 = \frac{2800}{13} = 215.38$. The values of $\widehat{F}_A^{\text{EC}}(t)$ at the jump times $t = 2$ and $t = 6$ become

$$\widehat{F}_A^{\text{EC}}(2) = \frac{13}{2800} \times \frac{35}{1 \times \frac{65}{140}} = \frac{7}{20} = 0.35$$

$$\widehat{F}_A^{\text{EC}}(6) = \frac{7}{20} + \frac{13}{2800} \times \frac{30}{\frac{50}{100} \times 1} = \frac{49}{140} + \frac{39}{140} = \frac{22}{35}$$

Both numbers are indeed the same as the ones based on the Aalen-Johansen estimator from Section 2.3.

2.4.3.2   The PL form

To derive the weights, we use the empirical version of (2.11):

$$\widehat{h}_k(t_{(i)}) = \widehat{P}(T_k = t_{(i)} | T_k \geq t_{(i)})$$

$$= \frac{\widehat{P}(T_k = t_{(i)})}{\widehat{\overline{F}}(t_{(i)}-) + \sum_{t_{(j)} < t_{(i)}} \widehat{P}(T^\circ = t_{(j)})}.$$

We use the ECDF form (2.19) for $\widehat{P}(T_k = t_{(i)})$ and $\widehat{P}(T^\circ = t_{(j)})$. For $\widehat{\overline{F}}(t_{(i)}-)$ a similar expression holds [37]:

$$\widehat{\overline{F}}(t_{(i)}-) = \frac{1}{\widehat{N}} \frac{r(t_{(i)})}{\widehat{\overline{T}}(t_{(i)}-) \times \widehat{\Phi}(t_{(i)}-)}. \tag{2.25}$$

The constant $\widehat{N}$ cancels and we obtain

$$\widehat{h}_k(t_{(i)}) = \frac{\dfrac{d_k(t_{(i)})}{\widehat{\overline{\Gamma}}(t_{(i)}-)\times\widehat{\Phi}(t_{(i)}-)}}{\dfrac{r(t_{(i)})}{\widehat{\overline{\Gamma}}(t_{(i)}-)\times\widehat{\Phi}(t_{(i)}-)} + \sum_{t_{(j)}<t_{(i)}}\sum_{l\neq k}\dfrac{d_l(t_{(j)})}{\widehat{\overline{\Gamma}}(t_{(j)}-)\times\widehat{\Phi}(t_{(j)}-)}} \tag{2.26}$$

$$= \frac{d_k(t_{(i)})}{r(t_{(i)}) + \sum_{t_{(j)}<t_{(i)}}\sum_{l\neq k}d_l(t_{(j)})\times\dfrac{\widehat{\overline{\Gamma}}(t_{(i)}-)\times\widehat{\Phi}(t_{(i)}-)}{\widehat{\overline{\Gamma}}(t_{(j)}-)\times\widehat{\Phi}(t_{(j)}-)}}. \tag{2.27}$$

The contribution of each individual to the denominator in (2.27) is equal to the weight $w_l(t_{(i)})$ as defined in (2.18). Note that $\widehat{\overline{\Gamma}}(t-)/\widehat{\overline{\Gamma}}(t_{(j)}-)$ decreases as time t increases, whereas $\widehat{\Phi}(t)/\widehat{\Phi}(t_{(j)}-)$ increases.

In Table 2.3 we show the calculations with the example data. $\widehat{\overline{\Gamma}}(t-)$ and $\widehat{\Phi}(t-)$ were calculated in Section 2.4.3.1. At 2 years, there were no competing events observed yet, hence $r^*(2) = r(2) = 100$. At 6 years, the observed number at risk $r(t)$ was 50. Forty individuals had a competing event at $t = 4$. Both $\widehat{\overline{\Gamma}}(4)$ and $\widehat{\Phi}(4)$ are equal to 1: no censorings had occurred yet, and there were no individuals that entered at a later time point. The censorings at $t = 5$ induce a weight of 0.5 at $t = 6$. Since $1 - \frac{65}{100} = \frac{35}{100}$ and $1 - \frac{13}{35} = \frac{22}{35}$, we obtain the same results as in the previous calculations.

TABLE 2.3
Detailed calculation of $\widehat{F_A}^{\text{PL}}(2)$ and $\widehat{F_A}^{\text{PL}}(6)$

	2 years	4 years	6 years
$\widehat{\overline{\Gamma}}(t-)$	1	1	0.5
$\widehat{\Phi}(t-)$	$\frac{65}{140}$	1	1
$d(t)$	35 (A)	40 (B)	30 (A)
$r^*(t)$	100		$50 + 40 \times \frac{0.5}{1} \times \frac{1}{1} = 70$
$\widehat{h_A}(t)$	$\frac{35}{100}$	0	$\frac{30}{70}$
$\widehat{F_A}^{\text{PL}}(t)$	$(1-\frac{35}{100}) = \frac{65}{100}$	$\frac{65}{100}$	$(1-\frac{35}{100})\times(1-\frac{30}{70}) = \frac{13}{35}$

If there is no censoring due to loss to follow-up we can use these weights as well, but we have an alternative. We know when the individuals that experienced a competing event would have been administratively censored. This has been called a situation with censoring complete information [34]. The estimator that uses the time of administrative censoring is not exactly equal to the one based on weights, and we no longer have the equivalence with the Aalen-Johansen estimator. However, the difference is likely to be small.

We can also think of a situation with "truncation complete" information. This occurs if we know the potential entry times for individuals that are missed because they had their event before they could enter the study. This may be rare, but a similar situation occurs when left truncation is a consequence of the presence of a time-varying variable or entry into a new state in a multi-state setting. In the example with calendar period of follow-up as covariable (Page 41), an individual that experienced a competing event in the first period would not be under observation in the second period, but he is not missed. We could think of an alternative estimator in which he is included in the risk set r^* from the moment at which he would have entered the second period onwards. We return to this in Section 5.3.3.

2.4.4 Interpretation of the weighted estimators

All nonparametric estimators that we have introduced can be derived via an algorithm that redistributes unobserved information as a consequence of left truncation and right censoring over observed individuals. In the PL and ECDF form, the redistribution is reflected by the presence of weights. But also the Aalen-Johansen estimator, with the Kaplan-Meier as a special case , can be derived in this way. We give a brief overview and make some further comments on the interpretation of the weights in the PL and ECDF form.

The Aalen-Johansen form

For the classical survival setting, the Kaplan-Meier has been derived using a "redistribution to the right" algorithm [30]. When an individual is right censored, his unobserved event time is equally redistributed over all the individuals that remain under observation. This idea can be extended to the competing risks setting, the only difference being that individuals that have a competing event are not treated as censored individuals [39]. The result is the Aalen-Johansen estimator. For its extension to left truncated data, the focus of the algorithm was changed: redistribution is done at each event time, and over all individuals that are under observation at that time [111].

The weight $\widehat{\overline{T}} \times \widehat{\Phi}$ in the PL and ECDF form

It has been suggested that the equivalence of the ECDF, PL and Aalen-Johansen form only holds if the censoring time C and the entry time V are independent [94]. Indeed, the product form of the weight is suggestive. If we do not have independence, the terms $1 - \frac{m_j}{r(c_{(j)})}$ and $1 - \frac{w_j}{r(v_{(j)})}$ in $\widehat{\overline{T}}(t-)$ and $\widehat{\Phi}(t-)$ estimate $P(C > c_{(j)} | C \geq c_{(j)}, V < c_{(j)})$ and $P(V < v_{(j)} | V \leq v_{(j)}, C > v_{(j)})$ respectively. If entry and censoring time are independent, the conditions $V < c_{(j)}$ and $C > v_{(j)}$ are superfluous and $\widehat{\overline{T}}(t-)$ and $\widehat{\Phi}(t-)$ estimate the time-to-censoring distribution and the time-to-entry distribution.

However, the equivalence between ECDF, PL and Aalen-Johansen estimator is an empirical relation, a relation that holds for any data set, irrespective of the underlying distributions. And the observed data do not allow us to determine whether entry time and censoring time are independent. We can use a similar graphical argument as was used in Section 1.5 for left truncated data: we only observe points in the lower right triangle of Figure 1.12, or even less if events prevent censorings to be observed, and we don't know the distribution of points in the upper left triangle. In fact, one could even argue that points in the upper left triangle cannot occur: how can we speak about censoring due to loss to follow-up, if the individual had not even entered the study? Yet, since we cannot conclude independence based on the data, we can always make the assumption if it helps to interpret the weights as estimators of the time-to-censoring and time-to-entry distributions.

The ECDF form

The ECDF form was first shown to be equivalent to the Kaplan-Meier for the situation with right censored data [88]. Later it was extended to the competing risks setting [111] and was also shown to be valid under both right censoring and left truncation [37].

The jump size in the ECDF form can be interpreted as an estimate of the probability that an event of type k occurs, given that the individual is under observation. Assuming that V and C are independent, we have

$$
\begin{aligned}
&\widehat{P}(T = t_{(i)}, E = k \mid V < t_{(i)}, C \geq t_{(i)}) \\
&= \frac{\widehat{P}(T = t_{(i)}, E = k, V < t_{(i)}, C \geq t_{(i)}))}{\widehat{P}(V < t_{(i)}, C \geq t_{(i)})} \\
&= \frac{d_k(t_{(i)})/\widehat{N}}{\widehat{T}(t_{(i)}-) \times \widehat{\Phi}(t_{(i)}-)}.
\end{aligned}
\tag{2.28}
$$

Note that $\widehat{N}$ is used, not N, because we estimate the probability over all individuals, also the unobserved ones.

The ECDF form can also be interpreted as the result of a redistribution of unobserved event times over the observed event time data. The difference with the algorithm that yields the Aalen-Johansen form is that mass is not equally redistributed but depends on $\widehat{T}$ and $\widehat{\Phi}$. Let $\widehat{p}_k(t_{(i)})$ be the jump size in the ECDF form at $t_{(i)}$ and let $\widehat{p}(t_{(i)}) = \sum_{e=1}^{K} \widehat{p}_e(t_{(i)})$. At any time t, an individual that is under observation also represents individuals that are missed because of left truncation: he is reweighted by an estimate of the probability to have entered the study by time t via $1/\widehat{\Phi}(t-)$. In our example data set we have $\widehat{\Phi}(2-) = 65/140$: an individual that is under observation at $t = 2$ is estimated to represent $140/65 = 2.15$ individuals (in reality 50% have entered by $t = 2$). An individual that is censored at $c_{(l)}$ has its mass redistributed over the individuals that have their event observed after $c_{(l)}$ according to

$$
\widehat{\pi}_k(c_{(l)}, t_{(i)}) = \frac{1}{\widehat{\Phi}(c_{(l)}-)} \times \frac{\widehat{p}_k(t_{(i)})}{1 - \sum_{j:t_{(j)} \leq c_{(l)}} \widehat{p}(t_{(j)})}.
$$

The individual that is censored at $c_{(l)}$ represents $1/\widehat{\Phi}(c_{(l)}-)$ individuals that are not observed, which induces the first term on the right-hand side. The second term is the probability, according to the $\widehat{F}_k$'s, to have an event of type k at later event times $t_{(j)}$, given that the censored individual was event free at $c_{(l)}$: $\mathrm{P}(T_k = t_{(i)} | T > c_{(l)})$.

Let $\widehat{\overline{\pi_k}}(t_{(i)}) = \sum_{l:c_{(l)} < t_{(i)}} \widehat{\pi_k}(c_{(l)}, t_{(i)})$ be the mass allocated to the observed event of type k at time $t_{(i)}$ from all the individuals that were censored at an earlier time point. Furthermore, let $\widetilde{d}_k(t_{(i)}) = d_k(t_{(i)})/\widehat{\Phi}(t_{(i)}-)$ denote the observed number of events of type k at $t_{(i)}$, again weighted for the missed individuals. It can be shown that the total probability of an event of type k allocated to $t_{(i)}$ via this redistribution mechanism is exactly equal to $\widehat{p}_k(t_{(i)})$ [37]:

$$\frac{\widetilde{d}_k(t_{(i)})}{\widehat{N}} + \frac{\widehat{\overline{\pi_k}}(t_{(i)})}{\widehat{N}} = \widehat{p}_k(t_{(i)}).$$

The constant $\widehat{N}$ can be seen as an estimate of the original sample size that includes the missed individuals. If we knew the size M of the sample that includes the missed individuals, $r(0+)/M$ would be an estimator of $\mathrm{P}(V \leq 0)$. We can use the observed number at risk $r(0+)$ because no events or censorings have occurred yet at $t = 0+$. Another estimator is $\widehat{\Phi}(0)$. Using relation (2.25) at $t = 0+$ and $\widehat{\overline{F}}(0) = \widehat{\overline{\Gamma}}(0) = 1$, we have $\widehat{\Phi}(0) = r(0+)/\widehat{N}$. Hence, $\widehat{N}$ can be seen to estimate M.

The PL form

In (2.26) we derived the estimator of the subdistribution hazard from the ECDF form. In Zhang *et al.* [111], another derivation of the PL form was given. Using (2.25), that weight is easily shown to be equivalent to the one from Section 2.4.3.2.

The interpretation of the ECDF form also applies to the PL form. Individuals with an event, of any type, are reweighted by the probability to be observed at their event time in order to account for events from unobserved individuals. Individuals that are observed to be at risk are reweighted by the same probability.

Another interpretation is based on (2.27), in which all the weights have been shifted to the individuals that had an earlier competing event. If we assume censoring and entry time to be independent, the censoring weight $\widehat{\overline{\Gamma}}(t_{(i)}-)/\widehat{\overline{\Gamma}}(t_{(j)}-)$ can be seen as an estimate of $\mathrm{P}\{C > t_{(i)} | C > t_{(j)}\}$, i.e. the probability that an individual remains free of censoring beyond the event time $t_{(i)}$, given that he was not censored when he experienced the competing event at $t_{(j)}$. Phrased otherwise: if we don't know when an individual that has a competing event at $t_{(j)}$ would have been censored, what we can do is to distribute his censoring time over the later observed censoring times according to the distribution $\widehat{\overline{\Gamma}}(t-)/\widehat{\overline{\Gamma}}(t_{(j)}-)$.

The truncation weights $\widehat{\Phi}(t_{(i)}-)/\widehat{\Phi}(t_{(j)}-)$ can be seen to correct for individuals that experienced a competing event before they would have entered the study. They are not observed, but ought to be included in the risk set because individuals remain in the risk set when a competing event occurs. They are represented by the individuals that had their competing event observed. At each event time $t_{(i)}$ of the type of interest, an individual that had a competing event observed at an earlier time point $t_{(j)}$ is still at risk. He represents individuals that had their competing event missed with a weight $1/\widehat{P}\{V < t_{(j)}|V < t_{(i)}\}$. The condition $V < t_{(i)}$ reflects that we calculate the risk set at $t_{(i)}$, the event $V < t_{(j)}$ reflects that this individual with the competing event at $t_{(j)}$ represents individuals that had a competing event at the same time but were missed. This weight is estimated by $\{\widehat{\Phi}(t_{(j)}-)/\widehat{\Phi}(t_{(i)}-)\}^{-1} = \widehat{\Phi}(t_{(i)}-)/\widehat{\Phi}(t_{(j)}-)$. Note that individuals that experienced the event of interest before they would enter the study are represented by the individuals that are observed to be at risk, as reflected in $r(t)$. For such individuals, no further correction is needed.

2.5 Standard errors and confidence intervals

In Section 1.8.2 we described the methods to estimate the variance of the Kaplan-Meier estimate and obtain pointwise confidence intervals around the curve. They are based on an estimate of the variance of the estimated cumulative hazard. In the competing risks setting, there are two hazards that can be used to estimate the cause-specific cumulative incidence. Each provides a different approach to quantify uncertainty in the estimate.

The multi-state approach

Most methods that have been suggested so far are based on the cause-specific hazard and the Aalen-Johansen estimator. In Braun and Yuan [16], estimators of the variance were summarized and their performance was compared in a range of simulation studies with data that were subject to right censoring only. The one that on average performed best was derived independently in papers by Gaynor *et al.* [35] and Betensky *et al.* [10]. Still, for small samples ($N \leq 50$), this Gaynor/Betensky estimator tended to be biased downwards. Later, the Gaynor/Betensky estimator was extended to the situation with left truncated data and was shown to be equivalent to the variance estimator from the multi-state setting that is based on the Greenwood-type variance estimator (1.16) of the cumulative cause-specific hazard [3]. It has a fairly complex structure that we don't repeat here (see e.g. Formula (6) in [3]).

Once we have an estimate of the variance $\widehat{\text{var}}\{\widehat{F_k}(t)\}$, we can use Formulas (1.20) and (1.22) from Section 1.8.2.1. Or we can use the ones from (1.23) that are based on $\widehat{F_k}(t)$ instead of $\overline{\widehat{F_k}}(t)$. With respect to performance, it is expected that the same holds as in the standard survival setting: the log scale is a good general choice, and the log-log scale may be preferred in small samples with few events ([15]). How the ones from (1.23) compare has not been studied. In Figure 2.8 we show the Aalen-Johansen estimate for SI as first event and the confidence intervals on the five different scales, using the `aidssi` data set (see Section 1.11.1). We zoom in on the first three years, where the differences are most pronounced; the estimate over the whole time range is shown in Figure 2.9. We observe that the linear scale and the log scale based on $\overline{\widehat{F_k}}$ are almost equal. The same holds for the log-log scale based on $\overline{\widehat{F_k}}$ and the log scale based on $\widehat{F_k}$. The log-log scale based on $\widehat{F_k}$ lies in-between.

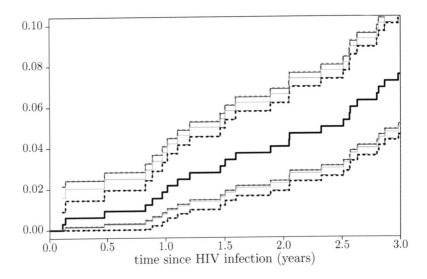

FIGURE 2.8
Comparison of different scales for calculation of 95% confidence intervals around estimate of SI-specific cumulative incidence. Dotted: log; solid: log-log; dashed: linear. Black: based on $\overline{\widehat{F_k}}$; gray: based on $\widehat{F_k}$

The subdistribution approach

Estimators of the variance can also be based on the subdistribution hazard and the product-limit estimator. The PL form has the same structure as the Kaplan-Meier and we can directly extend the approach for the Kaplan-Meier estimator to the competing risks setting. Using the delta method, the variance of $\widehat{F_k}^{\mathrm{PL}}$ is estimated as

$$\widehat{\mathrm{var}}\left\{\widehat{F_k}^{\mathrm{PL}}(t)\right\} = \{\widehat{F_k}^{\mathrm{PL}}(t)\}^2 \times \widehat{\mathrm{var}}\left\{\widehat{H_k}(t)\right\}.$$

Similar to Section 1.8.2.1, we define two variance estimators for $\widehat{H}_k$

$$\text{Aalen:} \quad \widehat{\text{var}}\left\{\widehat{H}_k(t)\right\} = \sum_{t_{(j)} \leq t} \frac{d_k(t_{(j)})}{\{r^*(t_{(j)})\}^2} \tag{2.29}$$

$$\text{Greenwood:} \quad \widehat{\text{var}}\left\{\widehat{H}_k(t)\right\} = \sum_{t_{(j)} \leq t} \frac{d_k(t_{(j)})}{r^*(t_{(j)})\{r^*(t_{(j)}) - d_k(t_{(j)})\}} \tag{2.30}$$

Confidence intervals on the log and log-log scale are based on Formulas (1.19) and (1.21).

In Figure 2.9 we plot the confidence intervals for SI as the first event using the Gaynor/Betensky and the PL-based estimator. Although they are not equivalent, they are visually indistinguishable.

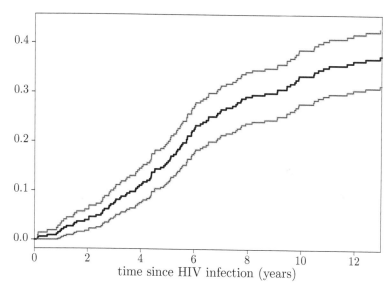

FIGURE 2.9
Estimate of SI-specific cumulative incidence and 95% confidence intervals on the log scale (1.20). Gaynor/Betensky: thick grey line; PL form: thin solid black line.

A more formal comparison with the Gaynor/Betensky estimator has been published in a Master's thesis [73], repeating the simulation studies A to D from Braun and Yuan [16]. Based on 1000 generated data sets, the average of the variance estimates was compared with the empirical variance, i.e. the variance of the 1000 estimates of the cause-specific cumulative incidence over the simulated data sets. Similar to the classical survival setting, the Greenwood-type estimator performed better than the Aalen-type. In Figure 2.10 results are summarized for the Greenwood-type estimator. We show the average value of the variance estimates relative to the empirical variance. The first column repeats the data generation for the four scenarios in the original paper (i.e. only right censored data). Results for the Gaynor/Betensky estimator varied slightly compared to the results in the Braun paper, which must be due to sampling variation. The subdistribution estimator of the variance was always larger than the Gaynor/Betensky estimator and tended to be closer to the empirical variance. We also investigated the effect of additional left truncation. With light truncation, i.e. 8% to 15% entering late, both estimators were very similar. With heavy truncation, i.e. 45% to 65% entering late, the subdistribution estimator was always smaller, and the Gaynor/Betensky estimator clearly performed better.

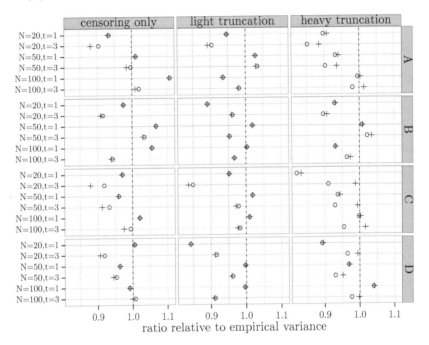

FIGURE 2.10

Comparison of variance estimators based on the Aalen-Johansen and the product-limit form. Method: $\widehat{F}_k^{AJ} = +$; $\widehat{F}_k^{PL} = \circ$.

Although the subdistribution approach performed well in the simulated data, no formal proof has been given yet with respect to its asymptotic performance. The martingale based approach as suggested in [37] may not be correct [65]. In fact, the Master's thesis also describes an example in which the Gaynor/Betensky estimator clearly outperforms the PL-based estimator, also for large sample size. This example is characterized by complete separation: all competing events happen first, next 30% of the remaining individuals is censored after which the event of interest occurs.

2.6 Log-rank tests and other subgroup comparisons

In Section 1.8.3 we described nonparametric tests for equality of time-to-event distributions in the classical survival setting. The most frequently used one, the log-rank test, is in essence a non-parametric test for equality of the corresponding (marginal) hazards. In the competing risks setting, we have two hazards and we can formulate a log-rank test for both.

The log-rank test for equality of the cause-specific hazards is the same as the log-rank test from the classical survival setting. This is because the nonparametric estimator of the cause-specific hazard is the standard hazard estimator. If all competing events are independent, it additionally tests for equivalence of the marginal hazards and marginal cumulative distributions. Since it has no one-to-one relation with the cumulative scale, it does not test whether the cause-specific cumulative incidences are the same.

If we want to use a nonparametric test for equality of cause-specific cumulative incidence functions, we can use the log-rank test based on subdistribution hazards, which does have the one-to-one correspondence with the cumulative scale. This test was first introduced by Gray [40] for right censored data. If k is the cause of interest, he defined a weighted number at risk for group g as

$$r_\omega^{(g)}(t_{(j)}) = r^{(g)}(t_{(j)}) \frac{\widehat{\overline{F_k}}^{(g)}(t_{(j)}-)}{\widehat{\overline{F}}^{(g)}(t_{(j)}-)}. \tag{2.31}$$

$r^{(g)}$ is the observed number at risk in group g, $\widehat{\overline{F_k}}^{(g)}$ is the group-specific Aalen-Johansen estimator of cause-specific cumulative incidence and $\widehat{\overline{F}}^{(g)}$ is the group-specific Kaplan-Meier estimator of overall survival.

$r_\omega^{(g)}$ is equal to the extended number at risk $r^{*(g)}$ with the weights based on the product-limit forms of $\widehat{\Gamma}$ and $\widehat{\Phi}$ from Section 2.4.2. This follows from relation (2.12) between cause-specific hazard and subdistribution hazard, applied to the distributions as defined by the estimators:

$$\frac{d_k(t_{(i)})}{r(t_{(i)})} \times \widehat{\overline{F}}(t_{(i)}-) = \frac{d_k(t_{(i)})}{r^*(t_{(i)})} \times \widehat{\overline{F_k}}(t_{(i)}-).$$

Therefore, Gray's statistic can be extended to left truncated data.

Define $r_\omega^{(\cdot)}(t_{(j)}) = \sum_g r_\omega^{(g)}(t_{(j)})$. For two groups, Gray's test statistic has the following form

$$Z^* = \sum_{j=1}^n K(t_{(j)}) \left[\frac{d_k^{(1)}(t_{(j)})}{r_\omega^{(1)}(t_{(j)})} - \frac{d_k(t_{(j)})}{r_\omega^{(\cdot)}(t_{(j)})} \right]. \tag{2.32}$$

With $K(t) = W(t)r_\omega^{(1)}(t)$, it can be rewritten as

$$\sum_{j=1}^{n} W(t_{(j)}) \frac{r_\omega^{(1)}(t_{(j)}) r_\omega^{(2)}(t_{(j)})}{r_\omega^{(1)}(t_{(j)}) + r_\omega^{(2)}(t_{(j)})} \left\{ \widehat{h_k}^{(1)}(t_{(j)}) - \widehat{h_k}^{(2)}(t_{(j)}) \right\},$$

which is the subdistribution equivalent of (1.26). Hence, the test statistic is a weighted difference between the group-specific estimates of the subdistribution hazard. The log-rank test is obtained when choosing $W(t) \equiv 1$.

Since $r_\omega^{(g)}$ is equal to $r^{*(g)}$, it can be calculated using group-specific $\widehat{\overline{\Gamma}}^{(g)}$ and $\widehat{\Phi}^{(g)}$. An alternative is to calculate one overall $\widehat{\overline{\Gamma}}$ and $\widehat{\Phi}$. Although the equivalence with Gray's test statistic is lost, the difference will be small as long as $\widehat{\overline{\Gamma}}$ and $\widehat{\Phi}$ do not differ much over the groups.

Another issue is the estimation of the variance of the test statistic. We can use the formula from the standard log-rank test, replacing $r(t)$ by $r^*(t)$. In the Master's thesis [73], it was shown that this approach is equivalent to the one suggested in [58], but differs from the one used by Gray. The performance of both approaches was compared in a simulation study similar to the one in Gray's paper [73]. In general, the difference between the approaches was small. Gray's variance estimator performed clearly better in the scenario with complete separation of the distributions that was mentioned at the end of Section 2.5.

As an example, we look at the effect of CCR5 genotype on both SI and AIDS as the first event. We test for both the cause-specific hazard and the subdistribution hazard. In Table 2.4 we give the p-values. For AIDS as the first event, both hazards differ significantly by value of CCR5. For SI as the first event, there is no significant difference by value of CCR5, but p-values are quite different.

TABLE 2.4
P-values log-rank tests for effect of CCR5 genotype

hazard type	AIDS	SI
cause-specific	1.9×10^{-5}	0.28
subdistribution	2.9×10^{-4}	0.94

A different effect on both hazards for SI is also seen when we plot the cumulative hazards by value of CCR5 (Figure 2.11). The cumulative cause-specific hazard for the wild type is consistently higher than the one for the CCR5-Δ32 deletion, whereas the curves for the cumulative subdistribution hazards cross around 10 years after HIV infection. We return to this difference in Section 5.2. Note that the cumulative cause-specific hazard is steeper than the cumulative subdistribution hazard (see exercise 2 in Section 2.8).

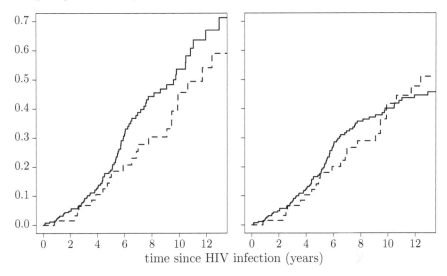

FIGURE 2.11
Estimated cause-specific (left panel) and subdistribution (right panel) cumulative SI-specific hazard. Solid lines: wild type CCR5. Dashed lines: CCR5-Δ32 deletion.

Alternatives to the log-rank tests

Gray's test is not very sensitive to nonproportional subdistribution hazards. Alternatively, we can extend tests that have been developed for the classical survival setting to the competing risks setting [62, 66]. An example is the Kolmogorov-Smirnov type test that compares the maximum difference between the estimates of the cause-specific cumulative incidences [68]. In [8], several procedures were summarized and compared with respect to type I error and power.

2.7 Summary; three principles of interpretability

In this chapter, we formally defined the theoretical concepts that were summarized in Table 1.1 on Page 15. In Table 2.5 we summarize the nonparametric estimators of these quantities. For the cause-specific cumulative incidence we developed three estimators.

The Aalen-Johansen estimator $\widehat{F}_k^{AJ}$ combines the Kaplan-Meier estimator of the overall cumulative incidence with an estimator of the cause-specific hazard. The cause-specific hazard is estimated in the standard way: individuals

TABLE 2.5

Estimators of hazard and cumulative incidence

hazard	estimate	cumulative
marginal[1]	$d_k(t)/r(t)\{= \widehat{\lambda}_k(t)\}$	$\prod_{t_{(j)} \leq t} \left\{ 1 - \widehat{\lambda}_k(t_{(j)}) \right\}$
cause-specific	$\widehat{\lambda}_k(t) = d_k(t)/r(t)$	$\widehat{F}_k^{\mathrm{AJ}}(t) = \sum_{t_{(j)} \leq t} \widehat{F}^{\mathrm{PL}}(t_{(j)}-)\widehat{\lambda}_k(t_{(j)})$
subdistribution	$\widehat{h}_k(t) = d_k(t)/r^*(t)$	$\widehat{F}_k^{\mathrm{PL}}(t) = \prod_{t_{(j)} \leq t} \left\{ 1 - \widehat{h}_k(t_{(j)}) \right\}$
	$\widehat{p}_k(t_{(j)}) = \dfrac{d_k(t_{(j)})/\widehat{N}}{\widehat{\Gamma}(t_{(j)}-)\,\widehat{\Phi}(t_{(j)}-)}$	$\widehat{F}_k^{\mathrm{EC}}(t) = \sum_{t_{(j)} \leq t} \widehat{p}_k(t_{(j)})$
overall	$\widehat{h}(t) = d(t)/r(t)$	$\widehat{F}^{\mathrm{PL}}(t) = \prod_{t_{(j)} \leq t} \left\{ 1 - \widehat{h}(t_{(j)}) \right\}$

[1] Only estimable if progression to the competing events is independent

leave the risk set when they experience a competing event. As a consequence, the estimate is often interpreted as a marginal hazard, which is not correct if censoring due to the competing risks is informative. On the other extreme, it has been suggested that it is never possible to estimate the marginal hazard in the presence of competing risks. Although censoring due to competing risks is often informative, there are situations in which the competing risk strikes at random. Death from a meteorite crash is a competing risk, but it does not invalidate a marginal analysis and make the estimates uninterpretable. And discharge from the hospital in Example 1.2.1 may be a noninformative competing risk of staphylococcus infection. But if we interpret the estimate as a marginal hazard, we should use the Kaplan-Meier estimator, not the Aalen-Johansen estimator, for the marginal cumulative incidence.

The product-limit estimator $\widehat{F}_k^{\mathrm{PL}}$ resembles the classical Kaplan-Meier. The estimator of the marginal hazard is replaced by an estimator of the subdistribution hazard. It differs from the estimator of the cause-specific hazard in the definition of the risk set. An individual that experiences a competing event remains in the risk set $r^*(t)$ until the time at which he would have been censored had he not experienced the competing event. If all censoring is administrative we know this censoring time[3]. A general approach is to estimate the time-to-censoring distribution and use it to predict the unobserved censoring time via multiple imputation or weights. We described the latter approach in detail. If there is left truncation, individuals that experienced their competing event before they would become at risk ought to be included in the risk set. In order to correct for these missed individuals, we use a weight based on the estimated time-to-entry distribution.

---

[3]The same holds in simulation studies.

The ECDF estimator $\widehat{F}_k^{\text{EC}}$ circumvents the use of hazards. It directly estimates the cause-specific cumulative incidence as a weighted frequency of observed events of the type of interest. The weights have the same structure as in the estimator of the subdistribution hazard.

Although they look very different, the AJ form, PL form and ECDF form are algebraically equivalent if we choose the weight function from Section 2.4.2. The same idea of censoring and truncation weights can be used for parameter estimation in a regression model for the subdistribution hazard or the cumulative incidence. If the censoring or entry time distribution depends on covariables that also affect the event-time distribution, then we need to make the weights depend on these covariables. We return to this in Chapter 5.

Standard errors and confidence intervals are usually based on the Aalen-Johansen form. They can also be based on the product-limit form. The latter method is easy to apply and seems to perform well in many situations.

If we want to investigate whether the hazards differ by group, we can use a log-rank test. Each type of hazard gives rise to a log-rank test.

Marginal hazards This is the log-rank test from the classical survival analysis setting. It also tests for equality of marginal cumulative incidences. It assumes that all truncation and censoring, also from the competing risks, is noninformative.

Cause-specific hazards This is the log-rank test from the classical survival analysis setting, but with a different interpretation. It does not require independence between the competing risks. Results cannot be translated to the cause-specific cumulative incidence.

Subdistribution hazards Also known as Gray's test. It also tests for equality of cause-specific cumulative incidences.

We have only discussed nonparametric estimation using data that may be subject to right censoring and left truncation. If the end point is interval censored, both nonparametric estimation as well as calculation of standard errors and confidence intervals become much more difficult [42].

Three principles of interpretability

We reflect upon three principles that have been formulated to judge interpretability of the estimand or model under consideration [5]:

1. Do not regard individuals as at risk after they have died
2. Stick to this world
3. Do not condition on the future

The subdistribution hazard violates the first criterion. However, there are situations in which an interpretable rate is obtained when individuals that are no longer at risk remain included in the risk set. One example is in the evaluation of the effect of vaccination for hepatitis B on infection rates over calendar time. If we exclude individuals from the risk set once they have been vaccinated, then we estimate the hepatitis B infection rate among susceptible individuals. A decrease in this infection rate over time is explained by increased herd immunity, i.e. a decrease in the number of infectious source individuals. If we do not remove the vaccinated individuals from the risk set, we quantify the trends in infection rate at the population level. A decrease in this rate not only reflects a decrease in the number of infectious source individuals but also a decrease in the number of susceptibles.

Another situation in which individuals can remain in the risk set is when the competing event is not observed directly. Individuals may no longer be susceptible to the event of interest because they are immune or cured. For example, individuals that are cured by cancer therapy are no longer at risk of relapse. Cure is not observed; we only observe that some individuals don't have a relapse. If we keep these individuals in the risk set, then we quantify the overall effect of the treatment on relapse rate. If we want to disentangle effects for cured and non-cured individuals and restrict to the individuals that are not cured, we are using what is commonly called a cure model [98, 76, 75]. Such models are often hard to fit because of insufficient information on cure.

The marginal hazard in the presence of competing risks violates the second criterion. Individuals that are censored administratively or that are or lost to follow-up can experience the event of interest. However, if an individual experiences a competing event, occurrence of the event of interest is completely hypothetical. Mathematically a joint distribution of all competing event times can be defined; this has been called the latent failure time approach to competing risks. However, the interpretation of the distribution in this hypothetical world in which all other competing events are removed may be awkward. We return to this issue in Section 6.

The pattern-mixture parametrisation of competing risks violates the third criterion. Instead of jointly modeling the combination (T, E), it splits the probability $P(T = t, E = k)$ into $P(T = t|E = k)P(E = k)$ [63]. We will only know the probability of experiencing an event of type k, $P(E = k)$, at the end of the time scale. In the same spirit is the vertical modeling parametrisation $P(E = k|T = t)P(T = t)$ [74]. However, the vertical modeling parametrisation does not violate the third principle and can be useful in practice.

The weight $\widehat{\Phi}$ seems to violate the third principle, because it is a product over all the later time points. However, $\widehat{\Phi}$ can be replaced by $N\widehat{\Phi}$ and the latter is only based on earlier time points [37].

2.8 Exercises

1. In Figure 2.11 we saw that the estimate of the cumulative cause-specific hazard is steeper than the estimate of the cumulative subdistribution hazard. Is this a general property?

2. Comment on this interpretation of cause-specific hazard

> We want to compare the cancer event rates in the virtual situation when the competing risks did not exist. The analysis of the cause-specific hazard models the event of interest in the absence of competing risk events and thus is the appropriate method.

3.* In (2.3) on Page 60 we derived that the sum of the cause-specific hazards equals the overall hazard. Is the overall hazard also equal to the sum of the subdistribution hazards?

4. Comment on the following statement

> When there are no competing risks, a log-rank test is used to compare Kaplan-Meier cumulative incidence curves. In competing risks settings, this test is inappropriate.

5. In Figure 1.15 we have seen that the Kaplan-Meier curves to death for IDU and MSM differed considerably. We explained why these results should not be interpreted as a difference in marginal cumulative incidence to AIDS. What can you say about the difference in cumulative cause-specific hazards between both groups?

6.* Show that the ECDF form is equivalent to the Aalen-Johansen estimator in the situation with complete follow-up.

7.* Let $F_1(t)$ denote the cause-specific cumulative incidence, with cause-specific hazard denoted by $\lambda_1(t)$. Let $\overline{F}(t)$ denote the overall survival, with corresponding hazard $h(t)$. As estimators we use $\widehat{\lambda_1}(t_{(i)}) = d_1(t_{(i)})/r(t_{(i)})$ and $\widehat{h}(t_{(i)}) = d(t_{(i)})/r(t_{(i)})$. What do the following statistics estimate?

$$\widehat{A_1}(t) = \sum_{t_{(j)} \leq t} \left[\prod_{t_{(k)} < t_{(j)}} \{1 - \widehat{h}(t_{(k)})\} \right] \widehat{h}(t_{(j)})$$

$$\widehat{A_2}(t) = \sum_{t_{(j)} \leq t} \left[\prod_{t_{(k)} < t_{(j)}} \{1 - \widehat{\lambda_1}(t_{(k)})\} \right] \widehat{\lambda_1}(t_{(j)})$$

$$\widehat{A_3}(t) = \sum_{t_{(j)} \leq t} \left[\prod_{t_{(k)} < t_{(j)}} \{1 - \widehat{h}(t_{(k)})\} \right] \widehat{\lambda_1}(t_{(j)})$$

8. In a study on long-term effects of treatment in childhood cancer survivors [106], the end point of interest was symptomatic cardiac event (CE). Death from other causes (DOC) was a competing risk. Analysis was restricted to persons that survived the first five years after diagnosis. In Figure 2.12, the estimate of the CE-specific cumulative incidence is compared with the Kaplan-Meier curve for CE as end point. The cause-specific cumulative incidence curve for DOC is shown as well.

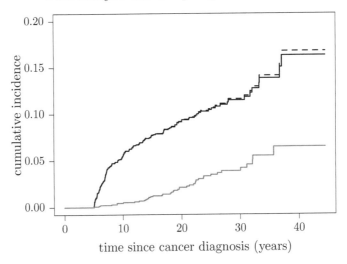

FIGURE 2.12
Estimate of CE-specific cumulative incidence (black solid line), Kaplan-Meier (dashed line) and DOC-specific cumulative incidence (gray line).

We see that the Kaplan-Meier (on the complementary scale of the cumulative incidence) and the estimate of the CE-specific cumulative incidence are almost equal. Comment on the following statement

> Death that is not caused by symptomatic cardiac events may not be related to having symptomatic cardiac events. In this case, ignoring the informative censoring mechanism does not substantially influence the estimates of symptomatic cardiac events.

9. In a study on the effect of gender on time from diagnosis of bladder cancer to relapse, death from other causes (DOC) was a competing risk. In Figure 2.13, we observe a strong effect of gender on relapse to both end points. One may wonder whether the lower risk of relapse for males may be explained by the higher mortality from other causes: the larger number of deaths among men prevents relapse to occur. In Figure 2.14, we plot both the Kaplan-Meier for relapse, in which individuals that die from other causes leave the risk set, and the estimate of relapse-specifc cumulative incidence estimate.

Comment on the following statement:

> The gender difference is also present in the Kaplan-Meier curves. Moreover, for both genders the cause-specific cumulative incidence function and the Kaplan-Meier are almost the same. Hence, the difference in relapse risk by gender cannot be explained by the larger competing death rates for males.

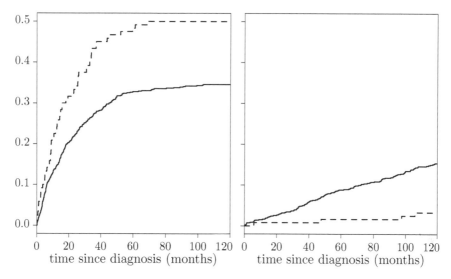

FIGURE 2.13

Estimate of cause-specific cumulative incidence for relapse (left panel) and death (right panel) for females and males. Solid lines: males. Dashed lines: females.

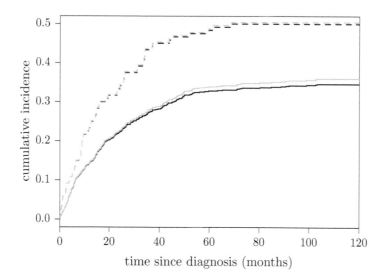

FIGURE 2.14

Estimate of relapse-specific cumulative incidence (black lines) and Kaplan-Meier (grey lines) for males (solid lines) and females (dashed lines).

2.9   Software

Estimation of the cause-specific hazard only uses techniques from classical survival analysis. Therefore, any program for analysis of time-to-event data can be used. The same holds for the log-rank test to compare cause-specific hazards. We concentrate on software to calculate the cause-specific cumulative incidence (Section 2.9.1) and software to test for differences between cause-specific cumulative incidences (Section 2.9.2).

An overview of packages for competing risks analysis in R is given in the section "Multistate Models" of the CRAN Task View on survival analysis[4]. A competing risks model is a special type of multi-state model. Therefore, the packages in the subsection "General Multistate Models" can also be used in the competing risks setting. The subsection "Competing risks" refers to packages that have been written specifically for competing risks situations.

2.9.1   Nonparametric estimation of F_k

Calculation of the nonparametric estimator of the cause-specific cumulative incidence and its confidence intervals is often based on the Aalen-Johansen form (2.14). It requires special code, which is explained in Section 2.9.1.1. An alternative is the product-limit form based on the subdistribution hazard. In the rare situation that we have complete or censoring complete information, we can use standard software to estimate the subdistribution hazard by redefining the risk set: an individual is in follow-up until either the event of interest or his (potentially unobserved but known) censoring time. If part of the censoring times is unknown, we can perform multiple imputation with the R package kmi. The alternative is to use weights. In Section 2.9.1.2 we explain in detail how to calculate the weights and use them in a weighted product-limit form.

2.9.1.1   The Aalen-Johansen form

In Stata, the estimate can be obtained via the stcompet command [25]. It uses the Gaynor/Betensky estimator of the variance. In SAS, the macros CUMINCID or %CIF can be used[5].

We describe two ways to compute the Aalen-Johansen form in R: 1) as implemented in the standard package for survival analysis, survival, 2) using the etm package. prodlim has similar functionality. One can also use packages that have primarily been written for multi-state models, such as mstate and msSurv that are explained in Section 3.7. In both survival and etm, the basic event time and status information is specified via the Surv function. We explained its structure for the classical survival analysis setting in Sec-

---

[4]See http://cran.r-project.org/web/views/Survival.html.
[5]See http://support.sas.com/resources/papers/proceedings12/344-2012.pdf

tion 1.11.2. In the competing risks setting, the specification of the event type differs between both packages. We use the `aidssi` data set as example (see Section 1.11.1 for a description of the variables).

The `survival` package

The `Surv` function has an argument `type`. If it is given the value `"mstate"`, then the time and status variables are interpreted as competing risks data and the Aalen-Johansen estimator is computed[6]. The variable that is specified in the `event` argument can have more than two values and can be of type numeric or factor. If it is a numeric variable, then the lowest value is assumed to represent censored observations. For example, if we use the `status` variable in the `aidssi` data set to specify the event types, the value 0 is interpreted as censoring. We can compute the estimate via:

```
csiSurv <- survfit(Surv(time=time,event=status,type="mstate")~1,
                                                    data=aidssi)
```

If the variable that is specified in the `event` argument is of class *factor*, then the `type` argument is assumed to have the value `"mstate"` by default. If we use the **cause** column, we can write

```
survfit(Surv(time=time,event=relevel(cause,"event-free"))~1,
                                                    data=aidssi)
```

Note that the lowest level of the factor is assumed to represent censorings. Since `AIDS` is the lowest level, we need to redefine it.

We obtain a detailed numeric description of the estimates using the `summary.survfitms` function[7]

```
summary(csiSurv, times=seq(2,10,by=2))
```

Its output resembles the one from `summary.survfit`. We show the values at five time points.

time	n.risk	n.event	prevalence1	prevalence2
2	300	15	0.00632	0.0404
4	240	52	0.10322	0.1112
6	170	54	0.17070	0.2259
8	122	41	0.25430	0.2916
10	81	32	0.33505	0.3346

The columns `prevalence1` and `prevalence2` give the estimates $\widehat{F_k}$ for the first (AIDS) and the second cause (SI) respectively. No standard errors and confidence intervals are shown, but they have been computed. They can be obtained by selecting the respective components of the output of the `survfit.formula`

---

[6]The former approach was by specifying the `etype` argument in the `survfit` function.

[7]This function does not have a help file, but it has the same functionality as `summary.survfit`.

or `summary.survfitms` function, e.g. `csiSurv$std.err`, `csiSurv$lower` and
`csiSurv$upper`. You are asked to do this in the computer practicals. Standard
errors are based on the Gaynor/Betensky estimator. By default, confidence
intervals are computed on the log-scale as specified in (1.19) on Page 35. The
scale can be changed via the `conf.type` argument in `survfit.formula`.

Results can be plotted using the `plot.survfit` and `lines.survfit` functions. The only difference from the classical setting is that `fun="event"` is the
default. For a plot on the survival scale, as in the alternate display format,
one specifies `fun="identity"`.

The *etm* package

The etm package[8] has a function `etmCIF` that calculates the Aalen-Johansen
estimator. After the package has been loaded into our R session we can use

```
csiEtm <- etmCIF(Surv(time=time,event=status!=0)~1, data=aidssi,
                                etype=status, failcode=c(1,2))
```

The `Surv` function is used in the classical way: the `event` argument only allows
to specify whether the individual had an event, of any type, or was censored.
The `etype` argument in `etmCIF` specifies the column that contains the event
type information. The `failcode` argument allows us to specify the end points
for which we want the estimates.

Results are summarized via `print.etmCIF` or `summary.etmCIF`.

```
summary(csiEtm)
```

gives as output

```
CIF 1
        P    time        var    lower   upper n.risk n.event
  0.00000  0.112 0.0000000 0.00000 0.0000    329       0
  0.08685  3.707 0.0002553 0.06039 0.1241    250       1
  0.17070  6.018 0.0004661 0.13282 0.2179    170       0
  0.32306  9.585 0.0007697 0.27209 0.3808     91       0
  0.40820 12.999 0.0008936 0.35232 0.4693     40       0
  0.41804 13.936 0.0009548 0.36025 0.4811      1       0


CIF 2
        P    time        var       lower    upper n.risk n.event
  0.00304  0.112 9.211e-06 0.0004287 0.02138    329       1
  0.09812  3.707 2.805e-04 0.0700299 0.13663    250       0
  0.22944  6.018 5.832e-04 0.1860947 0.28100    170       1
  0.31857  9.585 7.478e-04 0.2683438 0.37554     91       0
  0.37523 12.999 8.524e-04 0.3210117 0.43532     40       0
  0.58196 13.936 9.548e-04 0.5222651 0.64291      1       1
```

---

[8]etm stands for "empirical transition matrix".

The estimates are shown in column `P` and the confidence intervals in `lower` and `upper`. Information is only given at some selected time points[9].

If we want the information at all time points, we need to extract it from the result of the `summary.etmCIF` function. The output is a list, in which the first component contains the estimates. The first component itself is a named list, with one component per event type. The names are composed of `CIF` and the value of the event type, separated by a space. Hence, the estimates for the first event type are obtained via

```
summEtm <- summary(csiEtm)
summEtm[[1]][["CIF 1"]]
```

If we had defined the competing risks via the **cause** variable, then we would use "CIF AIDS" and "CIF SI":

```
summEtm <- summary(etmCIF(Surv(time=time,event=status!=0)~1,
          data=aidssi, etype=cause, failcode=c("AIDS","SI")))
summEtm[[1]][["CIF AIDS"]]
```

The result is a data frame with the same seven columns as above and a row for each unique time point with event or censoring.

The Gaynor/Betensky estimator of the variance is computed. Confidence intervals can be obtained on four scales. The default is `"cloglog"`, which is the complementary log-log scale as defined in (1.21) and (1.22) on Page 35. The complementary log-log scale (1.23) is specified via `"log-log"`. The value `"log"` uses the log scale in the form as specified in (1.23); the other log scale is not provided. The value `"linear"` uses the linear scale (1.18).

Another way to obtain information at all time points is via the functions `trprob.etm` for the estimate and `trcov.etm` for the variance. Both function have primarily been written to obtain estimates in multi-state models (see Section 3.7.1). In the first argument of both functions we specify the first component in the output of the `etmCIF` function[10]. We specify the end point on which we want the information via the argument `tr.choice`. Its value should be in the form of a transition, as is usual in multi-state models. For example, if SI is the end point of interest (transition from the intitial state 0 to state 2), we obtain the estimates via:

```
trprob(csiEtm[[1]], tr.choice="0 2")
trcov(csiEtm[[1]], tr.choice="0 2")
```

We ask for estimates at specific time points via the `timepoints` argument. Confidence intervals are calculated using any of the formulas from Section 1.8.2.1.

The etm package has special functions `plot.etmCIF`, `plot.etm` and `lines.etm` to plot the estimates, but they cannot be used to plot on the

---

[9]The quantiles 0, 0.25, 0.5, 0.75, 0.9, and 1 of ther combined event and censoring times.

[10]The output of the `etmCIF` function is of class *etmCIF*, whereas an object of class *etm* is required. The first component of the etmCIF output list is of class *etm*.

survival scale. For the confidence intervals, they allow for the same four scales as `summary.etmCIF`. If we want more flexibility, we can create a data frame with the estimates ourselves. This was done when creating Figure 2.8 (see the code in the file `ExampleCode.R` on the book's website).

2.9.1.2   The weighted product-limit form

To incorporate information on time-varying weights, we use the counting process representation as described on Page 41. We first explain how the weights $\omega_l(t)$ in (2.18) can be computed. Once we have added the weights to our data, we can use standard code that has been written for the Kaplan-Meier. The only requirement is that the code allows for probability weights.

Computation of the weights

Consider three example individuals from a larger data set as in Table 2.6. Each has a different end point; the first individual was censored, the second experienced the event type of interest 1 and the third had the competing event 2.

TABLE 2.6
Three example individuals

id	entry.time	event.time	event.type
1	0.25460	0.63644	0
2	0.00000	0.64358	1
3	0.08005	0.25615	2

In Table 2.7 we show the data set in a representation that includes the weights. The follow-up information for the first two individuals does not change: they are at risk with a weight of one from their entry time until they are censored or experience the event of interest. The first row of the third individual refers to his actual follow-up period, again with a weight of one. After the event he remains in the risk set with a weight that changes over time. It needs to be evaluated at all later event times of type 1. Every new weight evaluation generates a new row. Suppose that the first seven observed event times of type 1 after 0.25615 were at 0.31778, 0.37693, 0.38928, 0.46029, 0.50979, 0.64358, and 0.64724. These times are in the **Tstop** column. Since calculations are only made at the event times, as value in the **Tstart** column we can choose any value between the previous event time and the value in **Tstop**. We choose the previous event time. The weights are split over two columns. Column **weight.cens** contains the censoring weights $\{\widehat{\overline{\Gamma}}(\texttt{Tstop}-)/\widehat{\overline{\Gamma}}(t_{(j)}-)\}$; $t_{(j)} = 0.25615$ is his event time, i.e. the value of `Tstop` in his first row. Column **weight.trunc** contains the weights $\{\widehat{\overline{\Phi}}(\texttt{Tstop}-)/\widehat{\overline{\Phi}}(t_{(j)}-)\}$ that correct for left truncation. The censoring weights change value if there was a censored observation between two subsequent event times. For example, individ-

TABLE 2.7

Same three individuals with time-varying weights

id	Tstart	Tstop	status	weight.cens	weight.trunc	count	failcode
1	0.25460	0.63644	0	1.00000	1.00000	1	1
2	0.00000	0.64358	1	1.00000	1.00000	1	1
3	0.08005	0.25615	2	1.00000	1.00000	1	1
3	0.25615	0.31778	2	1.00000	1.02941	2	1
3	0.31778	0.37693	2	1.00000	1.02941	3	1
3	0.37693	0.38928	2	1.00000	1.02941	4	1
3	0.38928	0.46029	2	1.00000	1.02941	5	1
3	0.46029	0.50979	2	1.00000	1.02941	6	1
3	0.50979	0.64358	2	0.67849	1.07230	7	1
3	0.64358	0.64724	2	0.67849	1.07230	8	1
⋮	⋮	⋮	⋮	⋮	⋮	⋮	⋮

ual 1 was censored at 0.63644 which changes the censoring weight between the event times 0.50979 and 0.64358. If there are no censorings between two event times, the weights in **weight.cens** do not change. Similarly, there were late entries at 0.28737 and 0.56966 (from other individuals in the data). These cause **weight.trunc** to change value at the subsequent event times 0.31778 and 0.64358. Rows in which both columns do not change value can be collapsed without losing information. For example, the period from 0.25615 until 0.50979 can be represented by one row, with weights 1.0000 for **weight.cens** and 1.02941 for **weight.trunc**.

The **status** column copies the event status from the original data set. The **count** column counts the row number within individuals. Hence the row with **count** equal to 1 reflects the period when the individual was in actual follow-up. The **failcode** column specifies the cause of interest.

In Stata, the data set with time-varying weights can be computed via the stcrprep command. In SAS the macro %PSHREG can be used [60]. In R, we can compute the weights using the crprep function, which is contained in the mstate package. All three have similar functionality, but the SAS macro currently does not compute truncation weights. We explain the use of the crprep function.

Assume that the data set for which we showed the first three individuals in table 2.6 is called dataset in R. The crprep function can be specified as follows:

```
crprep(Tstop="event.time", status="event.type", data=dataset,
    trans=1, cens=0, Tstart="entry.time", id="id", shorten=FALSE)
```

The required arguments Tstop and status have as value the column names that contain the event times and event types. The values in trans (the event type of interest) and cens (the value to denote censored observations) are 1 and 0, which are the defaults. Hence, they can be left out. Since there is left

truncation, we specify the entry time via the `Tstart` argument. By default
it is assumed to be zero for every individual, which is the situation without
delayed entry. The `id` argument can be used if we want to keep the original
individual identifiers in the weighted data set. If this argument is not specified,
persons are given a number based on their row position in the original data
set. By default rows in which the weights do not change are collapsed. This
can be overridden via `shorten=FALSE`. Other variables can be copied to the
weighted data set via the `keep` argument.

We create the weighted data set from the `aidssi` data. The columns **status**
and **cause** give the same information on event type, but in a different format.
If we use the **cause** column we write

```
aidssi.w <- crprep("time", "cause", data=aidssi,
                   trans=c("AIDS","SI"), cens="event-free",
                   id="patnr", keep="ccr5")
```

Since there is no late entry, the `Tstart` argument is not specified. The `crprep`
function allows for the creation of the weighted data set for several event
types at once by specifying them in the `trans` argument. An alternative to
specifying the column names is to give the actual values in the respective
columns.

In Table 2.8 we show some rows from the output of the `crprep` function.
Since there is no left truncation, only a column **weight.cens** with censoring
weights has been created. The first 2756 rows represent the data set with
weights for `AIDS` as event of interest. These rows have the value `AIDS` in the
`failcode` column. Individuals with `SI` as first event remain in the risk set
with time-varying weights. An example is individual 8, who had an SI switch
at 8.605. Rows 2757 and further represent the data set in which `SI` is the event
of interest. Individuals 3 and 15, who had `AIDS` as first event, are reweighted;
we show their first three rows.

The weighted product-limit form

In Stata, the weights are included by specifying the `iweights` option in the
`stset` command. The product-limit form is calculated via the standard `sts`
command. In R, the standard `survfit.formula` function in the `survival`
package is used.

If we want the SI-specific cumulative incidence, we restrict to the rows
that have `failcode` equal to SI and use

```
survfit(Surv(Tstart,Tstop,status=="SI")~1, data=aidssi.w,
        weights=weight.cens, subset=failcode=="SI")
```

Since we have two time columns to represent the time updated weights, we
need to use the counting process specification. For the specification of the
status we use the logical statement `status=="SI"` (see Section 1.11.2). If
there had been additional left truncated data, the weights should have been
specified as `weights=weight.cens*weight.trunc`.

TABLE 2.8

The weighted `aidssi` data set as created by the `crprep` function

	patnr	Tstart	Tstop	status	weight.cens	ccr5	count	failcode
3	3	0.000	2.234	AIDS	1.000	WW	1	AIDS
17	8	0.000	8.605	SI	1.000	WW	1	AIDS
18	8	8.605	8.638	SI	0.991	WW	2	AIDS
19	8	8.638	8.755	SI	0.982	WW	3	AIDS
.	.	.	. .		.	.		
78	14	0.000	5.054	event-free	1.000	WW	1	AIDS
79	15	0.000	10.196	AIDS	1.000	WM	1	AIDS
			⋮					
2768	3	0.000	2.234	AIDS	1.000	WW	1	SI
2769	3	2.234	2.322	AIDS	0.997	WW	2	SI
2770	3	2.322	2.982	AIDS	0.993	WW	3	SI
.	.	.	. .		.	.		
2870	8	0.000	8.605	SI	1.000	WW	1	SI
2913	14	0.000	5.054	event-free	1.000	WW	1	SI
2914	15	0.000	10.196	AIDS	1.000	WM	1	SI
2915	15	10.196	10.448	AIDS	0.974	WM	2	SI
2916	15	10.448	10.467	AIDS	0.961	WM	3	SI

We can also obtain the estimates for both end points at once by writing

```
csiPL <- survfit(Surv(Tstart,Tstop,status==failcode)~failcode,
                              data=aidssi.w, weights=weight.cens)
```

The specification ~`failcode` calculates estimates per value of `failcode`, i.e. for both end points separately. This specification is similar to the computation of the Kaplan-Meier per value of CCR5 on Page 56. Per value of `failcode`, the event of interest occurs when the `status` variable has the same value as the `failcode` variable, as specified in the logical statement `status==failcode`.

Characteristics of each of the two estimates can be selected via square brackets, in which we define the value of `failcode` that we want. For example, we select the information with respect to SI as event type at 2, 4, 6, 8 and 10 years using

```
summary(csiPL["failcode=SI"],times=seq(2,10,by=2))
```

and obtain

```
time n.risk n.event survival std.err lower 95% CI upper 95% CI
   2    302      13 0.959615  0.0110     0.938344     0.981369
   4    272      22 0.888783  0.0177     0.854687     0.924239
   6    218      34 0.774112  0.0240     0.728466     0.822619
   8    190      18 0.708440  0.0265     0.658364     0.762324
  10    161      11 0.665410  0.0279     0.612936     0.722377
```

Instead of `csiPL["failcode=SI"]`, we can also use the ordering of event types as assumed by the `survfit.formula` function. One way to learn this ordering is by looking at the `strata` component of the output:

```
csiPL$strata
failcode=AIDS    failcode=SI
        310             310
```

We see that SI is the second event type and we can write `csiPL[2]`. Standard errors are based on the subdistribution approach. In Figure 2.9 we compared the confidence intervals based on the multi-state and the subdistribution approach and noticed that they were almost equal.

2.9.2   Log-rank tests

The log-rank test for equality of cause-specific hazards can be performed with the standard log-rank test. In R we use the `survdiff` function. For SI as end point we write

```
survdiff(Surv(time,status==2)~ccr5, data=aidssi)
```

and obtain

```
n=324, 5 observations deleted due to missingness.

           N Observed Expected (O-E)^2/E (O-E)^2/V
ccr5=WW 259       84     79.2     0.290      1.15
ccr5=WM  65       23     27.8     0.827      1.15

 Chisq= 1.1  on 1 degrees of freedom, p= 0.284
```

Cause-specific cumulative incidence functions can be compared using Gray's log-rank test. In SAS, we can use the `%CIF` macro. In R, the `cmprsk` package has implemented Gray's test. After this package has been loaded we can test for a difference in progression to SI and AIDS by CCR5 genotype via

```
with(aidssi, cuminc(time, status, group=ccr5)$Tests)
```

and obtain

```
           stat           pv df
1 13.149851204 0.0002875421  1
2  0.005817877 0.9392003078  1
```

The first rows is the test result for cause 1, i.e. AIDS, the second for SI.

An alternative is to first create the extended data set with time-varying weights and perform the log-rank test based on the extended number at risk r^*. If there is no specific code to perform such a log-rank test, we can use the equivalent score test from a proportional subdistribution hazards model with the group as single covariable. In Stata, we fit a proportional subdistribution hazards model using the `stcrreg` command (see also Section 5.7.2).

We show how to perform the log-rank test in R using the data set with time-varying weights. We calculate group specific weights via the `strata` argument in `crprep`:

```
aidssi.wCCR <- crprep("time", "cause", data=aidssi,
        trans=c("AIDS","SI"), cens="event-free", strata="ccr5")
```

If we want to use one overall weight function we copy the `ccr5` column to the extended data set via the `keep` argument (see the computer practicals).

Since the data is in counting process format, the `survdiff` function cannot be used. We use the score test from the proportional subdistribution hazards model. The `coxph` function can incorporate time-varying weights in the same way as the `survfit.formula` function does. We need to distill the value of the test statistic and calculate the p-value ourselves.

```
test.AIDS <- coxph(Surv(Tstart,Tstop,status=="AIDS")~ccr5,
                data=aidssi.wCCR, weights=weight.cens,
                    subset=failcode=="AIDS")
test.SI <- coxph(Surv(Tstart,Tstop,status=="SI")~ccr5,
    data=aidssi.wCCR, weights=weight.cens, subset=failcode=="SI")
## score test statistic and p-value
## AIDS
c(test.AIDS$score, 1-pchisq(test.AIDS$score,1))
[1] 12.428139562  0.000422913
## SI
c(test.SI$score, 1-pchisq(test.SI$score,1))
[1] 0.007207246 0.932344471
```

We see that the results are comparable to Gray's test as implemented in the `cmprsk` package.

The packages `surv2sample` and `CIFsmry` can be used to test directly on the cause-specific cumulative incidence.

2.10 Computer practicals

In Section 1.12 we looked at event-free survival. Now we will study each event type separately. The exercises use some extra variables that have been added to the `ebmt1` data set in Exercise 2 in Section 1.12.

1. **Estimation** Estimate the cause-specific cumulative incidence for relapse and relapse-free mortality. Save the results in an R object. What is the probability, with 95% confidence intervals on one of the log scales, to have a relapse within one year and within five years. Try approach (c) based on the weighted product-limit form and at least one of the two approaches that use the Aalen-Johansen form, (a) or (b).

1. (a) *Using standard code in the* **survival** *package.* Have a look at the help file of the **Surv** function. Pay special attention to what is described about the **mstate** value in the **type** argument. Use the **survfit** function.

2. (b) *Using the etm package.* You may first have to install the package from some R server. Have a look at the help file of the **etmCIF** function.

3. (c) *Using the weighted product-limit form.* Use the **crprep** function to create the data set with weights. Have a look at its help file.

   Store the data set as an object named **Webmt1**. Include the covariables **score** and **age** and also store the **type** column in the new data set. Compute the weights for both end points.

   Inspect the first ten rows of the weighted data set that contain information for each of the two end points. What do the newly created variables represent? How many rows does the newly created data set have?

Compare the estimates with the relapse-free survival distribution, i.e. the probability to remain free of both event types.

2. **Some plots** We make some plots, using either of the approaches from Exercise 1.

(a) Plot the estimated cause-specific cumulative incidence for each end point using the overlaid display format. Plot the 95% confidence intervals on the scale of your choice.

(b) Plot the estimated cause-specific cumulative incidence using the stacked format (without the confidence intervals). First plot the relapse-specific cumulative incidence, and plot the death-specific cumulative incidence on top of this curve.

(c) Plot the cause-specific cumulative incidence estimates for each end point using the alternate display format. You can leave out the confidence intervals.

3. **Effect of EBMT risk score** We investigate the effect of the EBMT risk score on the cause-specific cumulative incidence (the variable **score** in the data set).

Estimate the cause-specific cumulative incidence for each of the three EBMT risk scores and for both end points. Use the Aalen-Johansen form (i.e. approaches (a) or (b)).

Plot the estimates; use one plot window for relapse and another one for death. If you use approach 1.(b), you can use the **which.cif** argument in the **plot.etmCIF** function. If you use approach 1.(a), creating the desired plot is fairly involved; the code is given in the file **ComputerPracticalsHints.pdf** on the book's website.

What do you conclude with respect to the effect of the EBMT risk score. Are the effects proportional?

4. **Choice of the weight function in the product-limit form** If we want to calculate the product-limit form that is equivalent to the Aalen-Johansen form for each value of **score**, the weights based on the censoring distribution need to be calculated separately as well. Create a data set that has the score-specific weights and name it `Webmt.score`.

Make plots to compare the results with the curves when we use the same weights per value of EBMT score, as was created in the data set `Webmt1`. What do you conclude with respect to the choice of the weight function?

The statistic $\widehat{\overline{T}}$ can be interpreted as an estimate of the time to censoring distribution. Estimate and plot the time-to-censoring distribution for each value of **score**. Does the distribution depend on the value of the EBMT risk score? Does this observation correspond to the amount of dependence on the weight function in the estimate of the crude risk?

5. **Log-rank tests** Run and compare the three commands given below. Why is the output from the first and the second different, and what do these commands test? Why do the second and the third give the same value of the test statistic?

```
coxph(Surv(Tstart,Tstop,status==1)~score, data=
  subset(Webmt.score,failcode==1), weights=weight.cens)$score
coxph(Surv(Tstart,Tstop,status==1)~score,
        data=subset(Webmt.score,failcode==1&count==1))$score
survdiff(Surv(time,stat==1)~score,data=ebmt1)
```

3

Intermediate Events; Nonparametric Estimation

3.1 Introduction; multi-state models

In the life sciences there is little interest in what happens after death; death, of whatever type, is the final event. Other event types are not fatal, and follow-up can continue. In Chapter 2 we looked at SI switch and AIDS as first events after HIV infection. But AIDS can also occur after an SI switch and an SI switch can occur after AIDS. Death is the final event, but neither SI nor AIDS is a prerequisite for mortality[1]. We mention three reasons to investigate the occurrence of intermediate events on the pathway to some final event.

First, it can give information on etiological mechanisms. In Section 1.2.3 we described the disease process after bone marrow transplantation. Patients may acquire acute graft-versus-host disease (AGvHD), which increases short-term mortality. However, if they survive the first period they have a lower relapse rate of the cancer. This protective effect of the intermediate event AGvHD on relapse is explained by an immune reaction of the donor T-cells against the diseased bone marrow of the host.

Second, it is useful for prediction, the clinical objective. Individuals with a chronic disease are seen regularly over time. During follow-up, events may occur that change the individual's prognosis. Suppose an individual acquired AGvHD 60 days after bone marrow transplantation, her platelets recovered after 120 days, and she has had no further events until one year after the transplantation. This information enhances the estimated probability to survive relapse-free for two more years. Or suppose an individual has been HIV infected for two years and the HIV virus switches to SI phenotype. The switch changes the estimated probability of developing AIDS within the next three years. In both examples, updated prognosis may guide decisions with respect to treatment or monitoring frequency.

The third reason is more statistical in nature. In classical survival analysis, we need to know the origin of the time scale for every individual. Individuals that enter after the initiating event often have an unknown time origin; they are left censored with respect to the initiating event. They are often excluded

---

[1]Unless AIDS related mortality is the end point, which cannot happen before AIDS.

from analysis, although they may comprise a major part of the study sample and contribute information on the later stages of the disease process. If we can add them from their first observed state onwards, we estimate the distribution of time from the intitiating event until the final event making maximal use of the available data: individuals that are followed from the intiating event onwards contribute information on the earlier stages, whereas individuals with unknown time origin are followed during the later stages of the disease. For example, many HIV/AIDS cohort studies have a large fraction of seroprevalent individuals, i.e. individuals that entered the cohort study after HIV infection and with unknown time since HIV infection. CD4 T-cell count is an important marker of progression to AIDS. By using this marker to quantify disease stage, we can include seroprevalent individuals in our estimate of the time from HIV infection to AIDS and death [90].

A multi-state model quantifies event rates and event risks based on the history of events[2]. We mainly consider multi-state models that satisfy the Markov property. The Markov property entails that what happens next only depends on the current state, not on what happened before. Markov models are composed of, and combine components that belong to either a classical survival setting or a competing risks setting. For this reason, they are covered in this book. The added value of combining all these components into one multi-state model is that we can predict the probability to be in an intermediate state, taking into account that this state can also be abandoned. Typically, probability curves can go up and down (see Section 3.4.2 for some examples). Another reason to use a multi-state model is when we are interested in etiology and want to quantify the effect of covariables on all transition rates. We may gain in power if we consider the whole process in one analysis (see Chapter 4 and especially Section 4.5). Furthermore, a multi-state approach helps to obtain more tailored predictions of final events if the effect of intermediate events on the future disease course depends on individual characteristics (see Section 5.2.2).

In Section 3.2 we describe the structure of multi-state models, introduce the terminology and formally define the Markov model structure. In Section 3.3 we address data representation and nonparametric estimation. In Section 3.4 the use of Markov models is illustrated by example: we investigate what happens in HIV infected individuals after they develop AIDS or have an SI switch as first event.

If you are only interested in the competing risks setting you can skip most of this chapter. Only the `mstate` package that is explained in Section 3.7.3 is used when we compute predictions based on a cause-specific hazards model in Section 5.7.1. Yet, reading this chapter helps to see the Aalen-Johansen estimator in the competing risks setting in broader perspective and to understand why programs for Markov multi-state models can be used for computation of the cause-specific cumulative incidence.

---

[2]For this reason it is sometimes called event history analysis.

3.2 Main concepts and theoretical relations

3.2.1 Basic framework and definitions

A multi-state model consists of states and transitions between them that reflect the assumed disease mechanism. It is recommended to start by making a graphical representation of the model via a directed graph. Such a graph consists of nodes and arrows. The nodes denote the states and are usually drawn as rectangles; the arrows, also called edges, denote the transitions and describe the disease pathway. We have seen examples of directed graphs in Sections 1.2.2 and 1.2.3 when describing the sequence of disease states after HIV infection and after bone marrow transplantation. Every node represents a dichotomous event. If the event is categorical then the levels can be split over different nodes, as was done with the causes of death in Figure 1.4.

States that only have outgoing arrows are called initial states. Most models have only one initial state. Intermediate states, states that have both incoming and outgoing arrows, are also called transient states. States that only have incoming arrows are called final or absorbing states. A multi-state model in which the directed graph only contains forward arrows is called irreversible or acyclic.

The simplest multi-state model beyond the competing risks setting is shown in Figure 3.1. It consists of three states and only has forward arrows. It is often called an illness-death model because it provides a concise description of the process from the healthy state to death. In the healthy state, there are the competing events diseased and dead. In the diseased state there is only one event type: dead. If we want to allow for disease recovery, we can add an arrow from the diseased state back to the healthy state.

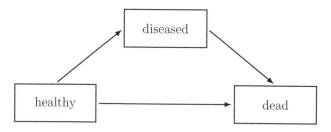

FIGURE 3.1
Graphical representation of illness-death model without recovery.

The directed graph only describes the possible transitions. In order to quantify rates and risks, we have to make further assumptions. The assumptions that we make depend on the suspected disease mechanism, but may also partly be determined by the amount of available data.

Although different graphs can be used to describe the same assumed disease mechanism, it is recommended to use a graph that directly reflects the assumptions that have been made. For example, suppose that we have recurrent events, such as in the illness-death model with disease recovery. If we impose a Markov structure and assume that the disease has no lasting effect, we add an arrow from the diseased state back to the healthy state in Figure 3.1: after recovery we are back in the same situation as before the disease. If we think that the first disease episode has an effect on subsequent disease recurrence, we obtain a clearer description if we add an extra recovery and disease state as shown in Figure 3.2.

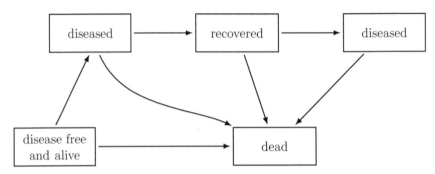

FIGURE 3.2
Graphical representation of acyclic illness-death model with disease recovery.

We can extend this figure with more recovery and disease states, but the amount of information may restrict the number of separate states in the model. There may be too few individuals that experience multiple disease episodes and we are not able to accurately quantify each transition separately. The problem of insufficient information is aggravated if we additionally want to quantify the effects of covariables on the transition rates, unless we assume these effects to be equal for certain transitions (see Chapter 4).

Usually, the process evolves in a patient time scale, in which entry into the initial state defines the overall time origin. However, each state that is reached can define another patient time scale: time since entry into that state. Which time scales are relevant depends on the biological mechanisms, the research aim and the assumptions that we wish to make in order to simplify estimation. An analysis in which all transitions are quantified with respect to the time since reaching the initial state is called a clock-forward approach. An analysis that resets the time origin every time a new state is reached is called a clock-reset approach.

In Section 3.4 we use a clock-forward approach because we think progression to AIDS and death is driven by time since HIV infection.

If we want to estimate the distribution of time from HIV infection to AIDS and death using states based on CD4 T-cell count, we use a Markov model with a clock-reset approach. We assume that CD4 is a surrogate marker for time since infection: what happens next only depends on the current state and the sojourn time spent in that state, not on time since HIV infection. Only in this way we can include seroprevalent individuals that have an unknown time of HIV infection.

We can also combine time scales. In patients with leukemia, diagnosis defines the overall time origin. If a patient receives a bone marrow tránsplant, his death risk is temporarily increased. Since patients receive a transplant at different times after diagnosis, the overall time scale cannot directly quantify the temporary change in mortality caused by the transplantation. We better add the time since transplantation as second time scale.

In the proportional hazards regression model, one time scale needs to be chosen as the principal one. The effect of other time scales can be quantified by including them as covariables in the model. An example is given in Section 4.5.4. A more coherent approach is to use a model in which all time scales are included as covariables [50].

Notation and theoretical relations

Classical survival analysis and competing risks are special cases of multi-state models. In the competing risks setting, there is one initial state from which at most one transition per individual can occur to a state $E \in \{1, \ldots, K\}$; in the classical survival setting we have $K = 1$. In a multi-state setting, individuals can start from different initial states from which they can move through a sequence of states. Let $\mathcal{X}^0$ be the set of initial states. If there is only one initial state, it is conveniently described as state 0. The whole disease process of an individual, during which period he is in which state, can be defined formally as a random process over time since the overall origin $\{X(t); t \geq 0\}$, with $X(t)$ taking values in $\{\mathcal{X}^0, 1, \ldots, K\}$. The complete state occupation history until time s is summarized as $\mathcal{H}_s = \{X(u); 0 \leq u \leq s\}$. An alternative description is via the event times and event types: $\{X^0, (T^1, X^1), \ldots, (T^L, X^L), \ldots\}$. $X^0 \in \mathcal{X}^0$ is the initial state, which can be left out if it is the same for everybody. $T^1 < T^2 < \ldots < T^L, \ldots$ denote the times of entrance into the states $X^1, X^2, \ldots, X^L, \ldots \in \{1, \ldots, K\}$. The process stops once an absorbing state is reached.

We can describe the randomness of the process via transition hazards or via cumulative probabilities. Again, in the presence of left truncation and/or right censoring, it is more convenient to use the hazard as a basis. For every state g, the transition hazard λ_{gh} to state h is the rate of progression to h as a subsequent state, given the history. For continuous distributions it is defined as

$$\lambda_{gh}(t) = \lim_{\Delta t \downarrow 0} \frac{P(X(t + \Delta t) = h \mid X(t) = g, \mathcal{H}_t)}{\Delta t}$$

Like all hazards, the transition hazard is an instantaneous probability, in this case to move to another state. Therefore, it is only defined for direct transitions. The cumulative transition hazard is defined as before. For continuous distributions it is the integral of the transition hazard, $\Lambda_{gh}(t) = \int_0^t \lambda_{gh}(s)ds$. For discrete distributions the integral is replaced by a sum.

The transition hazard generalizes the cause-specific hazard to the multi-state setting. In a competing risks setting, all transitions start from the same initial state and therefore there is no need to mention it explicitly in the notation. But if we would call it state 0, the cause-k specific hazard can be written as λ_{0k}.

Effects on the cumulative scale are described via transition probabilities. They are defined for any two states g and h and any two time points $s < t$ as the probability to be in state h at time t, given that one was in state g at time s and given the history $\mathcal{H}_s$:

$$\mathrm{P}_{gh}(s,t) = \mathrm{P}(X(t) = h \mid X(s) = g, \mathcal{H}_s).$$

$\mathrm{P}_{gh}(s,t)$ is zero if there is no pathway from g to h. With s fixed, $\mathrm{P}_{gh}(s,t)$ can go up and down over time t. It cannot decrease if h is an absorbing state that cannot be abandoned. The transition probability is also defined for $g = h$. Since an individual is always in some state, $\mathrm{P}_{gg}(s,t)$ is equal to $1 - \sum_{h \neq g} \mathrm{P}_{gh}(s,t)$. In an irreversible multi-state model, $\mathrm{P}_{gg}(s,t)$ is the probability to remain in state g between s and t. The transition probabilities for all pairs of states can be gathered into a transition matrix

$$\mathbf{P}(s,t) = \{\mathrm{P}_{gh}(s,t)\}. \tag{3.1}$$

The transition probability concerns two states. We can also define probabilities that characterize a single state. The state-g occupation probability is the prevalence of state g, $\mathrm{P}(X(t) = g)$. If everybody starts from the same initial state 0, it is the transition probability $\mathrm{P}_{0g}(0,t)$. The state-g entry distribution function is the probability to have been in state g by time t, irrespective of what happens next. A similar quantity is the state-g exit distribution function, the probability to have left state g by time t.

In a Markov model, the transition hazard and transition probability depend on the past only through the current state, not through the remaining history of the process. For the probability the Markov property entails

$$\begin{aligned}
\mathrm{P}_{gh}(s,t) &= \mathrm{P}(X(t) = h \mid X(s) = g, \mathcal{H}_s) \\
&= \mathrm{P}(X(t) = h \mid X(s) = g).
\end{aligned} \tag{3.2}$$

Such a model is completely determined by the transition hazards, just like a competing risks model. Unless specified otherwise, we assume that our model has the Markov property.

In a semi-Markov model, the transition probability depends on the current state and on how long ago it was reached. In a clock-reset approach, it becomes a Markov model which is called a Markov renewal process.

3.3 Estimation

3.3.1 Data representation

There are several ways in which we can represent the data on observed transitions. The initial data set is often in a wide format: all information from an individual is in one single row.

There are two wide data formats. In a *time-ordered* format, every observed transition generates two columns, one for the transition time and one for the state that is reached. The same representation was introduced on Page 109, except that part of the process may be unobserved due to late entry and right censoring. The data from an individual is $\{(v_i, x_i^0), (t_i^1, x_i^1), \ldots, (t_i^{L_i}, x_i^{L_i}), c_i\}\}$. v_i denotes the entry time; a column with that information is not needed if everybody is observed from the time origin onwards. If the first observed state is the same for every individual, the column with information on x_i^0 can be left out. If the last state that is reached is not absorbing, there may be extra follow-up in that state. Then c_i is needed to denote the total follow-up time. Typically, the number of transitions differs per individual. An individual with fewer observed transitions than the maximum per individual has empty columns after his last observed transition.

A *state-ordered* format can be used in irreversible multi-state models. Every possible state in the model generates two columns. One column contains the first observation time in that state and the other column is a zero-one variable that denotes whether the state was reached during follow-up. If an individual did not visit the state, his total follow-up time is used and the state column has the value of zero. Again, extra columns are used if the initial state or the entry time is not the same for all individuals.

For analysis, we usually need to transform the data set to a long format. In a long format, the information from one individual is split over several rows. In a *transition-based* format, there is one row per observed transition, plus one row for the last observed state in case of censoring (see Section 3.4). In a *stacked* format, there is one row per possible transition. Its naming and usefulness is clarified in Section 4.3.

3.3.2 Nelson-Aalen and Aalen-Johansen estimator

Before performing the analyses, the following considerations are important to reflect upon.

- *What do we want to estimate?* Options are 1) the (cumulative) transition hazard, 2) the transition probability, 3) the state occupation probability, 4) the state entry or exit distribution.

- *Which transitions or states are we interested in?* The transition hazard is only defined for direct transitions. Is one of the states of interest an initial or absorbing state?

- *Which time scales are relevant?* Do we use a clock-forward approach, a clock-reset approach or do we consider several time scales in one analysis?
- *What time points are we interested in?* For the transition probability, are we only interested in one combination of s and t, do we want to vary one of them or do we want to consider all combinations? If we fix s and vary t, we predict the future based on the history at s (*fixed history prediction*). If we fix t and vary s, we quantify how the prognosis changes with updated information as we get closer to the time t (*fixed horizon prediction*).

Before defining the estimators, we need to specify the assumptions with respect to right censoring and left truncation. Since individuals can pass through a sequence of states, the multi-state setting is more complicated. An individual is not censored for intermediate states that he is observed to have visited, but may be censored for later states. A definition that encompasses the whole multi-state process is to consider an individual right censored when his follow-up terminates before he has reached an absorbing state. State transitions that are not observed because he moved to competing states are not interpreted as censorings; they are part of the multi-state process. There is left truncation due to late entry if individuals are missed because they experienced an absorbing event before they would enter the study. Another form of left truncation occurs because intermediate states are reached after the time origin. Only from that moment onwards do individuals become at risk for the subsequent transitions. This internal left truncation [6]—see also Page 42—is seen as part of the process and not interpreted as late entry.

Often it is assumed that both distributions, right censoring and late entry, are completely independent of the multi-state process. The censoring time C_i has no relation with the states that have been visited, nor with the states that would be visited if the individual had remained in follow-up. And the fact that an individual enters the study in a certain state (usually the initial state) at time V_i is unrelated to the states that he has reached before entry, nor to the states that will be visited after entry. If he enters in a non-initial state he does have a history, but it has not influenced his probability to enter.

A slightly weaker assumption is that the censoring time is state dependent. This means that the distribution of the censoring time may change after the transition to another state. Since all quantities are defined relative to some current state, state dependent censoring can be assumed without loss of generality.

The transition hazard is estimated in the same way as the cause-specific hazard. Let $Y_g(s)$ be the number of individuals that is in state g at time s, i.e. is at risk for transitions out of g. If there are $d_{gh}(s)$ transitions from g to h observed at s, the estimate is

$$\widehat{\lambda_{gh}}(s) = \frac{d_{gh}(s)}{Y_g(s)} \ . \tag{3.3}$$

The Nelson-Aalen estimator of the cumulative transition hazard $\widehat{\Lambda_{gh}}(t)$ is the sum of the transition hazard estimates: $\widehat{\Lambda_{gh}}(t) = \sum_{s \le t} \widehat{\lambda_{gh}}(s)$.

The general procedure for estimation of transition probabilities in Markov models is the Aalen-Johansen estimator. It is based on the transition hazard. We first explain its structure for the irreversible illness-death model from Figure 3.1. Let the states 0, 1 and 2 refer to "healthy", "diseased" and "dead" respectively. Then we have

$$\widehat{P_{00}}(s,t) = \prod_{s < u \le t} \left\{ 1 - \widehat{\lambda_{01}}(u) - \widehat{\lambda_{02}}(u) \right\} \tag{3.4}$$

$$\widehat{P_{11}}(s,t) = \prod_{s < u \le t} \left\{ 1 - \widehat{\lambda_{12}}(u) \right\} \tag{3.5}$$

$$\widehat{P_{12}}(s,t) = \sum_{s < u \le t} \widehat{P_{11}}(s, u-) \widehat{\lambda_{12}}(u) \tag{3.6}$$

$$\widehat{P_{01}}(s,t) = \sum_{s < u \le t} \widehat{P_{00}}(s, u-) \widehat{\lambda_{01}}(u) \widehat{P_{11}}(u+, t) \tag{3.7}$$

$$\widehat{P_{02}}(s,t) = \sum_{s < u < t} \widehat{P_{00}}(s, u-) \widehat{\lambda_{01}}(u) \widehat{P_{12}}(u+, t)$$

$$+ \sum_{s < u \le t} \widehat{P_{00}}(s, u-) \widehat{\lambda_{02}}(u) \tag{3.8}$$

The probabilities for the backward transitions are zero.

We explain each of them. We take sums and products over u, but note that jumps can only occur at observed transition times. The right-hand side in (3.4) is nothing but the Kaplan-Meier estimator of the probability to remain in state 0, starting from s. Similar to the competing risks setting, the sum of the transition hazards from state 0 is the overall hazard. $\widehat{P_{11}}(s,t)$ in (3.5) is the Kaplan-Meier estimator of the probability to "survive" in state 1. $\widehat{P_{12}}(s,t)$ in (3.6) is equal to $1 - \widehat{P_{11}}(s,t)$, because state 2 is the only state that can be reached from state 1 and it is absorbing. We have formulated it more generally as a competing risks Aalen-Johansen estimator which also holds if there had been several absorbing states that could be reached from state 1.

The other two estimators have a structure that goes beyond the competing risks setting. A transition from state 0 at time s to state 1 at time t can be observed at any time u between s and t. The term $\widehat{P_{00}}(s, u-) \widehat{\lambda_{01}}(u)$ in (3.7) is the jump in the competing risks Aalen-Johansen estimator at an observed transition to state 1 at time u. The term $\widehat{P_{11}}(u+, t)$ takes into account that individuals should not have moved to state 2 between u and t. Because of this term, the estimator $\widehat{P_{01}}(s,t)$ can also decrease when t increases[3]. $\widehat{P_{02}}(s,t)$ in (3.8) combines the two possible pathways to move from state 0 at time s to state 2 before time t. All quantities are defined on earlier lines. Note that

---

[3]We have been a little bit sloppy in notation: if $u = t$, then $t+$ is larger than t, but then we define $\widehat{P_{11}}(t+, t) = 1$.

we write $s < u < t$ as the summation in the first term, because an individual cannot jump from 0 to 1 and from 1 to 2 at the same time.

$\widehat{P}_{12}(s,t)$ is also defined for $s = 0$. Since 1 is not an initial state, formally $\widehat{P}_{12}(s,t)$ only makes sense from some $s > 0$ onwards: individuals start to become at risk for the transition from 1 to 2 some time after the time origin. However, the estimate remains zero as long as s is smaller than the time of the first observed transition from 1 to 2.

Since individuals enter state 1 over time, the first transition from 1 to 2 may happen when there are very few individuals at risk in state 1. In the most extreme case, the first individual that enters state 1 moves to state 2 before any other individual has entered state 1. This will blow up our estimate of the transition probability and its derived quantities. In the example in Section 3.4, this occurs for the transition from AIDS/SI to death (see Figure 3.5). In such situations, it is better to estimate a conditional distribution, i.e. from a time point onwards at which there is a sufficient number of individuals at risk, as we do in Figure 3.6. The problem is less severe for the estimate of the cumulative transition hazard. In Figure 3.4, the jump size is one, but the estimate still makes sense at later time points when there are more individuals in state 1.

The general form of the Aalen-Johansen estimator can be written as a concise matrix product

$$\widehat{\mathbf{P}}(s,t) = \prod_{s < u \leq t} \left\{ \mathbf{I} + \widehat{d\Lambda}(u) \right\}. \tag{3.9}$$

$\widehat{\mathbf{P}}(s,t)$ is the matrix of transition probabilities (3.1). $\mathbf{I}$ is the identity matrix. $\widehat{d\Lambda}(u)$ is a matrix that has $\widehat{\lambda_{gh}}(u)$ as off-diagonal elements $(g \neq h)$; its elements along the diagonal are equal to minus the sum of all off-diagonal elements along the same row: $-\sum_{h \neq g} \widehat{\lambda_{gh}}(u)$. Detailed explanations of this formula can be found in many articles and books, see for example [1, 6, 7] or the original paper [2].

Since state occupation probabilities are transition probabilities from the intitial state, we can use the same Aalen-Johansen estimator. If there are no censored observations nor late entries, we can estimate the state occupation probabilities in a very simple way, similar to what was done in Section 2.4.1: we calculate the fraction of individuals that are in state h at time t. This direct estimation cannot be done for transition probabilities $P_{gh}(s,t)$ in general. The reason is that individuals enter state g at later time points, which induces (internal) left truncation.

The variance of the Aalen-Johansen estimator is estimated via the variance of the Nelson-Aalen estimator. For the latter, either the Aalen-based or the Greenwood-based estimator can be chosen (see Page 34). The transformation to the variance estimator of the transition probability is fairly complicated and left out here (we refer to e.g. [1, 6]). Confidence intervals can be calculated on different scales; the most commonly used ones were explained in Section 1.8.2.1.

The Aalen-Johansen estimator is only valid in Markov models. Estimation of transition probabilities for a clock-reset Markov renewal process has been discussed in [96]. Beyond these models, transition probabilities are much harder to estimate, but some suggestions have been made [72, 71]. Another option may be the inclusion of a frailty term to model unobserved heterogeneity that makes some individuals have higher transition hazards than others [82].

There is one exception. For estimation of state-occupation probabilities, the Aalen-Johansen estimator is also valid if the Markov assumption is not fulfilled [26]. The reason is that it quantifies a characteristic of the process from the time origin and the initial state onwards, hence there is no history on which to condition. The same holds for the Nelson-Aalen estimator, because it only concerns transitions out of a specific state. The only requirement is that right censoring and late entry are completely independent of the multi-state process. For state dependent censoring a generalisation using inverse probability weights has been suggested [27].

A simple way to estimate the state-g entry and state-g exit distributions in an irreversible multi-state model is by reducing it to a model in which g itself is an absorbing state (for the state-g entry distribution) or by creating an extra absorbing state that combines all outgoing transitions from state g.

3.4   Example: HIV, SI, AIDS and death

As an example, we study the disease course from HIV infection to death, with SI and AIDS as intermediate events. The possible transitions were given in Figure 1.5 in Section 1.2.2.

All individuals in the data set are men who have sex with men (MSM). In this group, mortality that is not AIDS-related is rare and we assume it to be independent (see also Table 1.2). Therefore we leave out the state "death, not AIDS related" and assume the structure in Figure 3.3.

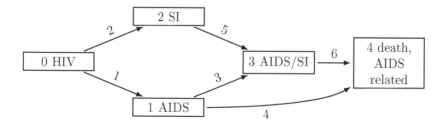

FIGURE 3.3
Directed graph of disease course from HIV infection to death, with SI and AIDS as transient states.

There is one initial state, there are three transient states and there is one absorbing state. From the initial HIV state and from state AIDS, there are two possible transitions; from the other states there is only one possible subsequent event type. We created a separate state for individuals that have switched to SI and developed AIDS. If we would use arrows between the states SI and AIDS, this would suggest that both events can occur more than once. We use one combined SI/AIDS state because of lack of data: only six individuals were observed to switch to SI after AIDS diagnosis. So we assume that, once an individual has switched to SI and developed AIDS, the sequence in which these events occurred is irrelevant for the progression rate to death (see also Exercise 2 in Section 3.6).

3.4.1   The data

We use the `aidssi2` data set that is contained in the R package `mstate`. It extends the `aidssi` data set in three ways. It contains information on what happened after the first event, it has age at infection as an extra variable, and it takes account of the fact that some individuals entered the study after HIV infection[4].

The `aidssi2` data set is in the state-ordered wide format. In Table 3.1 we show the complete information from the same four individuals as in Table 1.3, who each had a different sequence of events. Time is relative to the initiating event, HIV infection. The entry time is shown in the **entry.time** column. Since all individuals in our data set were first observed in the HIV state, there is no need to specify the initial state as a separate column. The columns **aids.time**, **si.time** and **death.time** give the transition times to the respective states. If a state was not reached, the time value represents the end of the follow-up for that individual. The columns **aids.stat**, **si.stat** and **death.stat** have the value 1 if these states were reached, otherwise they have the value 0. AIDS and SI can occur in any sequence.

TABLE 3.1

Time and status information from four individuals in the `aidssi2` data set

entry.time	aids.time	aids.stat	si.time	si.stat	death.time	death.stat
0.00	5.05	0	5.05	0	5.05	0
1.81	2.23	1	2.26	0	2.26	1
1.80	10.20	1	12.93	0	12.93	0
2.80	11.46	1	8.61	1	11.94	1
⋮	⋮	⋮	⋮	⋮	⋮

For estimation, we need to use one of the long formats. In Table 3.2 we show

---

[4]The left truncation has been ignored in the `aiddsi` data set for historical reasons: when the data set was first used, the weighting approach in competing risks analysis with left truncated data did not exist yet.

the information from the same four individuals as in 3.1 in the transition based long format. The stacked long format is shown in Table 4.5. The **patnr** column gives the personal indentifier from the `aidssi2` data set (which is just the row number). The **entry** column shows when the individual was first observed in the HIV state or when a transient state was reached. The state information itself can be read from the **from** column. The **exit** column shows when the individual was right censored or when the transition to another state occurred. The state information can be read from the **to** column. **entry** and **exit** give time with respect to the overall time origin, HIV infection. The **time** column gives the time that was spent in the respective states[5]. We additionally show the information on the CCR5 genotype and age at HIV infection.

TABLE 3.2
Time and status information in transition-based long format for the individuals from Table 3.1

	patnr	entry	exit	time	from	to	ccr5	age
28	14	0.00	5.05	5.05	HIV	cens	WW	34.9
4	3	1.81	2.23	0.43	HIV	AIDS	WW	39.0
5	3	2.23	2.26	0.02	AIDS	death	WW	39.0
29	15	1.80	10.20	8.40	HIV	AIDS	WM	26.8
30	15	10.20	12.93	2.74	AIDS	cens	WM	26.8
14	8	2.80	8.61	5.80	HIV	SI	WW	30.8
15	8	8.61	11.46	2.85	SI	AIDS/SI	WW	30.8
16	8	11.46	11.94	0.48	AIDS/SI	death	WW	30.8

In Table 3.3 we summarize some basic transition and state occupation characteristics. The first four columns show the observed number of transitions from the states as given in the row names to the states as given in the column names. The observed numbers are all between 80 and 120, except for the switch to SI after AIDS, i.e. the transition from AIDS to AIDS/SI, which was only observed six times. The column **no event** shows the number of individuals that was right censored. The column **total** shows the number of individuals that was observed to have visited the state as given by the row name.

3.4.2 Analyses

We choose a clock-forward approach because we see time from HIV infection as the driving force behind progression to AIDS. Hence, we use the time values in the columns **entry** and **exit** in Table 3.2. In a clock-reset approach we would use the **time** column. Inspired by the considerations on Page 111, we estimate several quantities and see what we can learn from them.

---

[5]Because of rounding to two digits, some numbers are not the same as the difference between **exit** and **entry**.

TABLE 3.3

Number of observed transitions (from row to column), number of censored observations and total number at risk

	SI	AIDS	AIDS/SI	death	no event	total
HIV	108	118	0	0	103	329
SI	0	0	89	0	19	108
AIDS	0	0	6	97	15	118
AIDS/SI	0	0	0	83	12	95

Cumulative transition hazard

We start with calculating the Nelson-Aalen estimates of the cumulative transition hazard. In Figure 3.4, the results are shown for all six direct transitions in overlaid format. The slope reflects the transition rate to the subsequent state. We observe that the two death rates are highest. The progression rate from SI to AIDS, the transition SI → AIDS/SI, is much higher than the rate of progression from HIV to AIDS. Hence the switch to SI is an unfavourable intermediate event.

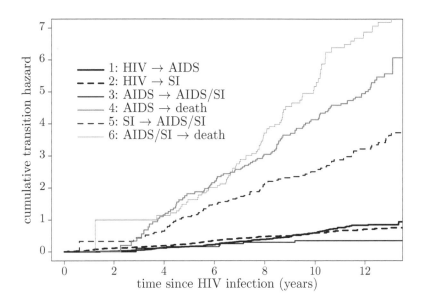

FIGURE 3.4

Nelson-Aalen estimates of the cumulative transition hazard for all six direct transitions.

For transitions that are not from the initial HIV state, individuals become at risk at later time points. Transitions may occur when few individuals are at risk. Indeed, this is observed for the transition from AIDS/SI to death: there is only one person at risk, resulting in a large jump from zero to one. For the other three transitions the number at risk at the first jump is larger, but still below 10 (Table 3.4). The number at risk increases thereafter, resulting in much smaller jump sizes and the slope becomes a more accurate estimate of the transition hazard. For the transitions HIV $\to$ SI and HIV $\to$ AIDS, the number at risk is large from the time origin onwards.

TABLE 3.4
Event time and number at risk at the first four transitions, stratified by transition type

1		2		3		4		5		6	
time	n	time	n	time	n	time	n	time	n	time	n
1.44	108	0.11	125	2.88	9	2.26	5	0.60	3	1.23	1
1.84	144	0.14	124	4.10	19	2.68	7	2.7732	19	3.70	7
2.16	291	0.47	121	6.19	20	2.91	9	2.7734	18	4.25	13
2.18	290	0.82	117	6.24	22	3.09	9	3.182	23	4.49	16

Transition probability, fixed history

The cumulative transition hazards out of a state do not translate directly to effects on the cumulative probability scale if there are competing transitions. We have seen this already in Chapter 2. In a multi-state setting there is the additional phenomenon that states can be abandoned. In Figure 3.5 we show the estimates of the transition probabilities $\widehat{P_{gh}}(0,t)$ for the same six transitions as in Figure 3.4. Since the transition probability combines all possible pathways, the transition AIDS $\to$ death not only comprises the direct transition, but also the one via AIDS/SI.

Because death is an absorbing state, the transition probabilities from AIDS and AIDS/SI to death cannot decrease. All other transitions are to transient states; these probabilities can go up and down and do not reach a high value. We overlay all estimates in one plot, but for a more detailed inspection of the transition probabilities to the transient states it is better to use a y-axis that only extends to the value 0.35.

The jump of size one in $\widehat{\Lambda_{gh}}(t)$ for the transition from AIDS/SI to death has a dramatic impact on the estimate of the transition probability: it jumps from zero to one and gives no information on the later part of the curve. The initial jump in the transition probability from SI to AIDS/SI is due to the same fast progressor. He had a switch to SI after 0.14 years and developed AIDS after 0.60 years. As can be seen from column 5 in Table 3.4, when he developed AIDS, there were 3 individuals in the SI state, hence the curve jumps to 0.33. Since he died before any other individual had moved from SI to AIDS/SI, the curve returns to zero and there is a new chance to get a meaningful estimate for this transition probability later on.

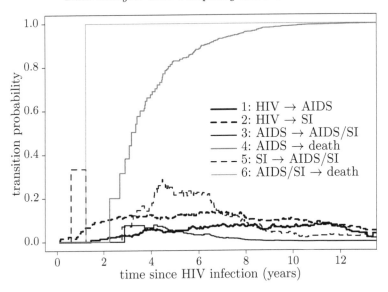

FIGURE 3.5
Aalen-Johansen estimates of the transition probability for all six transitions
with a direct path.

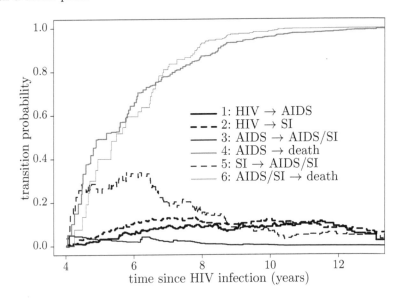

FIGURE 3.6
Aalen-Johansen estimates of the transition probability for all six transitions
with a direct path, from four years onwards.

We can prevent the large jumps in the beginning by estimating the transition probabilities from some later time point onwards. In Figure 3.6 we show the estimates $\widehat{P}_{gh}(4,t)$ from 4 years. From this figure we can observe that the death probability is not much influenced by the status with respect to SI after AIDS diagnosis: the transition probabilities for AIDS $\rightarrow$ death and AIDS/SI $\rightarrow$ death are similar.

In Figure 3.7 we plot the estimated state occupation probabilities $\widehat{P}_{0h}(0,t)$ for all five states. It can be seen that around 50% is expected to die within 10 years after HIV infection. The probability to be in any of the transient states is always smaller than 15%. The probabilities add up to the value one.

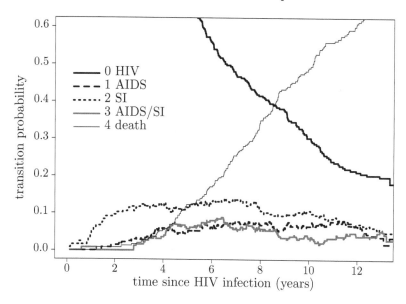

FIGURE 3.7
Aalen-Johansen estimates of all state occupation probabilities.

We can also estimate transition probabilities to combinations of states. Individuals with AIDS can be in two states, depending on whether the virus has switched to the SI phenotype. When estimating the probability to be alive with AIDS, we add the state occupation probabilities $\widehat{P}_{01}(0,t)$ and $\widehat{P}_{03}(0,t)$ for AIDS and AIDS/SI. The result is shown in Figure 3.8. We also show the 95% confidence intervals (CI), based on the Greenwood estimator and calculated on the log scale via Formula (1.20) on Page 35. We also plot the estimated probability to be in the state AIDS without SI, which was already shown in Figures 3.5 and 3.7. The difference between both curves is the probability to be in the state AIDS/SI.

When estimating the transition probability to an absorbing event, we can also ignore all intermediate events. As an example, we estimate the marginal distribution of time from HIV infection to death via the Kaplan-Meier and

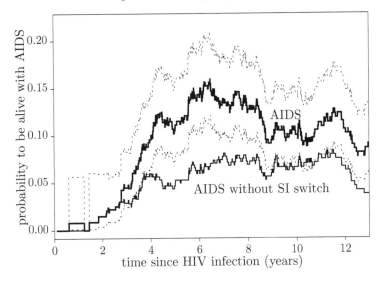

FIGURE 3.8
Probability to be alive with AIDS (thick solid curve), with 95% CI (dotted lines). Thin solid curve is estimated probability to be in state 1, AIDS.

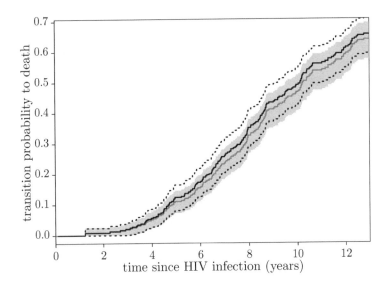

FIGURE 3.9
Distribution of time from HIV infection to death. Grey curve and area: Kaplan-Meier estimator, with 95% CI. Black lines: Aalen-Johansen estimator based on a multi-state model, with 95% CI.

compare this with the Aalen-Johansen estimator of $P_{04}(0, t)$. The result is in Figure 3.9.

The estimates are slightly different. The reason for the difference may be that the right censoring mechanism is state dependent. Then the Aalen-Johansen estimator is still valid if the Markov property holds, but the Kaplan-Meier is not. If the time-to-censoring is shorter for the later states, then the estimate of the cumulative incidence based on the Kaplan-Meier will be biased downwards: individuals that are censored are closer to the end point. Note that without right censoring and late entry both estimates would be the same.

Transition probability, fixed horizon

Until now we have quantified the future from a fixed time point s onwards ($s = 0$ or $s = 4$), the fixed history prediction. We can also quantify how the probability to be in some state at a fixed time point in the future changes as we get closer to that time point, the fixed horizon prediction.

In Figure 3.10 this is shown for two situations: if we are AIDS-free and without a SI switch (state HIV) and if we are AIDS-free but after a switch to SI (state SI). Of course, the closer we get to ten years, the more likely it is that we remain in our current state until the horizon. This is seen by the two curves that go up to the value 1, whereas all other curves go down to zero.

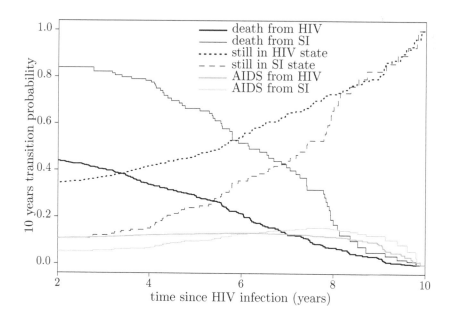

FIGURE 3.10
Fixed horizon prediction at ten years after HIV infection, starting in states HIV and SI.

We observe that the probability of having died by ten years is always higher if the virus has switched to SI, which again reflects that the switch to SI before AIDS diagnosis worsens the prognosis. The lower probability of remaining in the SI state, compared to the HIV state, reflects the same mechanism. For an HIV infected individual that has NSI virus type and is AIDS-free at some time between 2 and 8 years, the probability of being alive with AIDS at ten years is about 13%. If the virus has already switched to the SI phenotype, this probability goes up slightly from 2 to 8 years. Note that being alive with AIDS for the ones that are currently in state HIV comprises the states AIDS and AIDS/SI.

State entry and state exit distribution

As an example, we estimate the probability of developing AIDS over time. This is a state entry distribution, with the state defined by the combination of state 1, AIDS, and state 3, AIDS/SI. The estimate can be obtained by using a multi-state model in which states 1 and 3 are absorbing events. In Figure 3.3 we remove the transitions 3, 4, and 6. We can also connect transition 5 the state 1, AIDS, such that it becomes an illness-death model. In Figure 3.11 we plot the estimate and compare it with the probability of being alive with AIDS, which was shown already in Figure 3.8. Since individuals with AIDS are likely to die shortly after, the latter curve remains much lower. Similar to what we observed in Figure 3.9, the estimate of the marginal distribution of time to AIDS based on the Kaplan-Meier is slightly lower (result not shown).

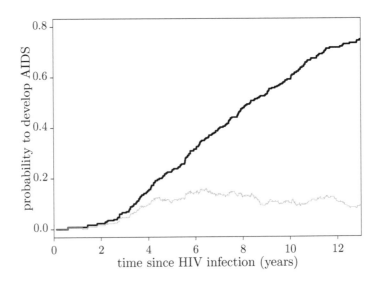

FIGURE 3.11

State-AIDS entry distribution (black) and the probability of being alive with AIDS (grey).

3.5 Summary; some alternative approaches

A multi-state model is used if we want to describe the sequence of events over time, if we want to quantify the prevalence of disease states over time, or if we want to predict how the occurrence of an event changes the disease course. It also has added value if we are interested in some final outcome, but censoring is state dependent.

The Nelson-Aalen estimator of the (cumulative) transition hazard has the simple form of a standard hazard estimator. It describes progression rates to subsequent states. It also forms the basis for the Aalen-Johansen estimator of the transition probability. The Aalen-Johansen estimator is only valid in Markov models, unless we restrict it to state occupation probabilities. Its computation is somewhat involved. In Section 3.7 we give suggestions for software. In Section 5.2.2 we discuss estimation of transition probabilities if the transition rates have been modeled to depend on covariables via a regression model. In Section 4.5 we describe one such regression model in detail: the proportional transition hazards model.

It is recommended to start by creating a transparent description of the basic structure of the process via a diagram with states that represent the event types and arrows that represent the possible transitions. Such a diagram is especially useful if the resulting multi-state structure has the Markov property. Then we can forget the past and zoom in on a specific state. If there are no backward transitions that can induce loops, such a diagram resembles a directed acyclic graph (DAG) that is used in causal inference. In a causal DAG, every arrow represents an assumed causal effect. A multi-state model can represent disease etiology as well, but its use is not restricted to the modeling of causal processes.

We only addressed the situation that all transitions have been observed exactly and with certainty. We did not consider interval censored transition times. With interval censored transition times we only observe state occupations at certain time points and do not know when the state was reached and whether the individual had been in other states since the last observation. We also did not consider misclassified states, which are often analyzed via hidden Markov models [17].

If we have recurrent events of the same type, it can be seen as a reversible multi-state model with two states. After each event, individuals can return to the intitial state and become at risk for the event again. This is in essence a classical survival analysis setting. However, there is often unobserved heterogeneity that makes some individuals have a higher event rate than others. We may be able to correct for this by including a frailty term. Another option is to use a robust sandwich estimator of the standard error [100].

Multi-state models are not the only approach used to describe disease mechanisms and make predictions based on updated information. We mention two alternative approaches, i) joint models for longitudinal and time-to-event data and ii) landmark models. Both approaches are more flexible with respect to the type of intermediate information. They can be used with any type of variable that changes over time, quantitative as well as categorical.

A joint model consists of two submodels, one for the longitudinal development of the disease characteristics, and one for the rate at which some final event occurs. The final event can be of more than one type as in a competing risks setting. In a selection model, the submodels are combined by making the event rate depend on the time-updated disease characteristics [84]. The disease characteristics can be either the measured values or the fitted values from the longitudinal model. In a pattern mixture model, the submodels are combined by making the longitudinal development depend on the final event time [101]. Joint models have a fairly complex structure and often several assumptions are made. But if the assumptions are correct, the model makes efficient use of the available data.

A landmark model can be used if we want to know how progression to the final event depends on time-updated disease characteristics. It incorporates time-updated information by choosing a sequence of points on the time scale, landmarks [108]. At each landmark, the final event time is regressed on the characteristics of the time-varying variables as known at the landmark. This can be done via a model on the hazard, but also via a model that quantifies effects directly on the cumulative scale, such as the proportional odds model (see Section 5.4). The models at the landmarks are often combined into one supermodel. Landmark models are attractive for their simplicity, but they do not model the development of the disease characteristics. Their effect on the event risk is quantified based on only time-fixed information known until the landmark.

3.6 Exercises

1. In the explanation of (3.6) for the transition from illness to death, we said that the Aalen-Johansen estimator is equivalent to the estimate based on the Kaplan-Meier. Why do we require the incoming death state to be absorbing in order for this equivalence to hold?

2. In a Markov model, the transition rate to a subsequent state only depends on the current state, not on the history. In the directed graph of our model (Figure 3.3), no discrimination is made with respect to progression to death between individuals that first had the SI switch and those that first developed AIDS. Draw the directed graph for a Markov multi-state model in which the transition rate from AIDS/SI to death is allowed to depend on the sequence in which SI and AIDS occur.

3. In the example from Section 3.4, we did not include a separate absorbing state for mortality that is not related to AIDS. It was assumed to be independent. Do the Nelson-Aalen estimator and the Aalen-Johansen estimator change if we had created another state for "death, not AIDS-related", without assuming that it was independent?

4. In Table 3.1 we showed the data on the example individuals 14, 3, 15 and 8 in the `aidssi2` data set using the state-ordered wide data format. What would the data look like in the time-ordered wide format?

5. In Figure 3.5 we plotted the transition probabilities for the direct transitions. Which ones can also be interpreted as state occupation probabilities?

6. Compare Figures 3.5 and 3.6. Why can the location and height of the peak for the transition from SI to AIDS/SI be different if we start at $s = 4$?

7. The estimate of the transition probability for AIDS $\rightarrow$ death as shown in Figures 3.5 and 3.6 not only comprises the direct transition, but also the one via AIDS/SI. How would we obtain the transition probability for the direct transition 4 only?

8.* In Figure 3.9 we see that both curves have jumps at the same time points. Can you explain this? In order to simplify the explanation, use an illness-death model as example and have a look at the structure of the estimators (3.4) to (3.8).

9.* In Figure 3.12 we plot the estimated transition probabilities from SI to death for different initial time points, $P_{25}(s_k, t)$, $s_k \in \{2, 3, 4, 5, 6, 7, 8\}$. We see that the curves never cross. Is this a general property?

3.7 Software

The Nelson-Aalen estimator of the cumulative transition hazard can be computed with standard software for survival analysis. For a specific transition $A \rightarrow B$, we create a data set in which an individual becomes at risk when he enters state A (see Section 1.8.5). For non-initial states A in the clock-forward approach, this requires the data to be presented in counting process format. If state B is reached from there, he has an event. He leaves the risk set if a transition to another state occurs first. Next, we fit a standard Cox model without any covariables. The baseline hazard from this null model is the estimate.

As an example, we compute the Nelson-Aalen estimate for the transition from state SI to state AIDS/SI. We use a data set that is in long transition-based format as in Table 3.2. We need to select the rows that represent individuals in the SI state (`from=="SI"`). The `to` column contains the information

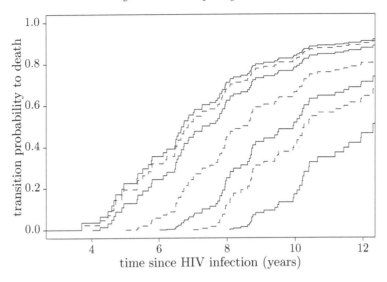

FIGURE 3.12
Estimate of probability to die over time for an individual in state SI at time $s_k = 2, 3, 4, 5, 6, 7, 8$ years.

whether the transition to AIDS/SI was observed. In R, if the data are in `data.trans`, we can use the following code

```
CumHaz.2to3 <- survfit(coxph(Surv(entry,exit,to=="AIDS/SI")~1,
                        data=subset(data.trans,from=="SI")))
```

In the stacked long format we can calculate the cumulative transition hazards for all transitions at once (see Section 3.7.3 and Chapter 4).

Computation of the Aalen-Johansen estimator of the transition probability is more involved. We do not know of any functionality in Stata or SAS. We explain three R packages that have been written for this purpose, `etm`, `msSurv` and `mstate`. Estimation in non-Markovian illness-death models has been implemented in the R package `TPmsm`. The `msm` package can be used if the transition hazard is assumed to be constant or piecewise contant over time. It allows for interval censored observations and misspecification of states via hidden Markov models. We refer to the section "Multistate Models" in the CRAN Task View on survival analysis for further options[6].

Table 3.5 summarizes the main options and requirements in `etm`, `msSurv` and `mstate` with respect to data structure and naming of variables. All three have the same basic functionality. The main advantage of the `etm` package is its ease of use for some standard procedures, like creating a plot of transition probabilities with confidence intervals in overlaid format. And it has some

---

[6]See `http://cran.r-project.org/web/views/Survival.html`.

TABLE 3.5

Nonparametric estimation in the R packages `mvna`, `etm`, `mSSurv` and `mstate`

	etm	mSSurv	mstate
specification			
transitions:	matrix, values TRUE and FALSE	create `graphNEL` object in `graph` package	matrix, values 1,2, ... and NA
data format :	long transition-based	long transition-based	long stacked
creation in R:	`etmprep`	use `etmprep` and adapt	`msprep`
estimation			
Nelson-Aalen:	`mvna`	via `mSSurv`	`msfit`
column names :	fixed, as in `etm`		flexible
state names:	flexible, character		1,2, ...
arguments:	`data` `state.names` `tra` `cens.name`[*]		`coxph` object `newdata`[*] `variance`[*] `vartype`[*] `trans`
Aalen-Johansen	`etm`	`mSSurv`	`probtrans`
column names	fixed:	fixed: **id start**[2]	flexible; `msprep`
in data set:	**id from** **to entry exit** **time**[1] created by `etmprep`	**stop** **start.stage** **end.stage**	creates **id** **from to trans** **Tstart Tstop** **time status**
state names:	flexible, character	flexible, character	1,2, ...
arguments:	as in `mvna` and `s` `t`[*] `covariance`[*] `delta.na`[*]	`Data` `tree` `cens.type`[*] `LT`[*] `bs`[*] `B`[*]	`msfit` object `predt` `direction`[*] `method`[*] `variance`[*] `covariance`[*]
results			
estimates:	`summary`	`summary`	`summary`
CI in `summary`:	`ci.fun`[*] `level`[*]	`ci.fun`[*] `level`[*]	
more flexible:	`trprob`	slots I.dA AJs ps or PSt SOPt	components of `probtrans`
(co)var :	`trcov`	slots cov.AJs var.sop or PSt SOPt	components of `probtrans`

[1]: in a Markov renewal process without left truncation we can use **time** instead of **entry** and **exit**

[2]: in a Markov renewal process without left truncation we can leave out **start**

[*]: optional argument

special functions for competing risks analysis. The `msSurv` package is the most flexible, but is more difficult to use in the beginning. In the `mstate` package it is easy to obtain numeric summaries and create a plot of transition probabilities from a specific state in any type of display format. Confidence intervals need to be calculated by the user based on the estimate of the standard error. It is easy to perform fixed horizon prediction and it has some special functions for competing risks analysis. It is the only package that computes transition probabilities based on proportional hazards regression models (see Sections 4.9 and 5.7). For all three packages a manual has been written that explains its basic use in more detail [4, 31, 28]. Here we concentrate on how the numeric results can be distilled from the computations, thus allowing the user to digest results with maximal flexibility. Since the Nelson-Aalen estimator forms the basis of the Aalen-Johansen estimator, it can also be computed with the code from these packages.

A program that computes the Aalen-Johansen estimate needs at least 1) the data with the observed state occupations and transitions, usually in a long format and 2) a specification of all allowed transitions. `etm` and `msSurv` require a transition-based format, whereas `mstate` requires a stacked format. The creation of the long data set can be done in a program of choice; `etm` and `mstate` have a special function to transform a wide state-ordered format to the required long format. The specification of the allowed transitions in `etm` and `mstate` is via a matrix with the number of rows and columns equal to the number of states in the model. The rows represent the outgoing states g and the columns represent the incoming states h; the cells specify whether a certain transition can occur. The values that need to be given in the cells differ between `etm` and `mstate` and are explained in Sections 3.7.1 and 3.7.3. The `msSurv` uses a special tree-like structure to define the model.

The `aidssi2` data set is in wide state-ordered format. It does not have separate columns for the "AIDS/SI" state. We need to create them ourselves; the R code can be found in the file `ExampleCode.R` on the book's website. We call these time and status columns **siaids.time** and **siaids.stat** respectively.

3.7.1   The `etm` package

Specify allowed transitions

The cells in the matrix that correspond to allowed direct transitions have the value `TRUE`, the others `FALSE`. Hence our 5-state model can be defined as

	HIV	AIDS	SI	AIDS/SI	death
HIV	FALSE	TRUE	TRUE	FALSE	FALSE
AIDS	FALSE	FALSE	FALSE	TRUE	TRUE
SI	FALSE	FALSE	FALSE	TRUE	FALSE
AIDS/SI	FALSE	FALSE	FALSE	FALSE	TRUE
death	FALSE	FALSE	FALSE	FALSE	FALSE

For clarity we have given state names to the rows and columns, but this is not required. We store this matrix in an object called `trans.etm`.

Create data set

We explain the use of the `etmprep` function to create the transition-based format. Its arguments resemble the ones in the `crprep` function which was explained in Section 2.9.1.2. It has as required arguments 1) `time`: a vector with the names of the columns that specify the transition (or censoring) times, one for every possible state, and given in the same order as in the transition matrix; 2) `status`: a vector of the same length as in 1) that has the names of the corresponding status columns; in each column, the value should be 1 if the state was reached and 0 if not; 3) `data`: the name of the data set; 4) `tra`: the matrix that defines the transitions.

The initial state is one of the states in the model and should be included in the vectors that are supplied to the `time` and `status` arguments. If the data set does not contain these columns, we can use `NA` as the column name. Before explaining the optional arguments, we first provide the code:

```
aidssi.etm <- etmprep(
  time=c(NA,"aids.time","si.time","siaids.time","death.time"),
  status=c(NA,"aids.stat","si.stat","siaids.stat","death.stat"),
  data = aidssi2, tra=trans.etm, cens.name="cens",
  state.names=c("HIV","AIDS","SI","AIDS/SI","death"),
  start=list(time=aidssi2$entry.time,
                          state=rep("HIV",nrow(aidssi2))))
```

The `cens.name` argument needs to be specified if there are censored observations. The value of `cens.name` is a character string that specifies how censored observations will be indicated in the long data format. It is recommended to specify the `state.names` argument as well; otherwise the states will be given names "0", "1" etcetera. Late entry is specified via the `start` argument. This argument does not accept column names; we have to provide the values of the entry times and the initial states via a list structure with components named `time` and `state`. All individuals in our data set started in state HIV; we create this vector on the fly. The `etmprep` also has an `id` argument which can be used if we want to keep the original values of the person indentifiers.

The computations

The Aalen-Johansen estimate is computed via the `etm` function. There is a corresponding package `mvna` that computes the Nelson-Aalen estimate via the `mvna` function. Both have a similar argument specification.

The first argument is the data set. The column names are required to be as specified in Table 3.5, i.e. **id**, **from**, **to**, **entry** and **exit**. In a Markov renewal process without left truncation, we can use one **time** column instead of the **entry** and **exit** columns[7]. The sequence in which the columns occur in the data set does not matter. The second required argument is the vector that defines the state names[8]. The other required arguments are the transition matrix and the starting value s from which we want to calculate the transition probabilities. If there are censored observations, the code for censored observations needs to be specified in the `cens.name` argument. If the optional argument t is not specified, the transition probabilities are calculated for all observed transition times $> s$. For the estimates in Section 3.4.2 we used

```
Prob.etm <- etm(aidssi.etm,
          state.names=c("HIV","AIDS","SI","AIDS/SI","death"),
          tra=trans.etm, cens.name="cens", s=0)
```

The increments of the Nelson-Aalen estimate are stored in the output as well, unless the argument `delta.na` is set to `FALSE`. For the computations that led to Figure 3.6 we used $s = 4$.

A fixed horizon prediction is more difficult to perform. We have to run the etm function for every value of s, while keeping t fixed.

Summarizing results via `summary.etm`

To obtain a numeric description of the estimates we can use the `summary.etm` function. Its output is a named list with one component per transition that has a direct path; the name is composed of the outgoing and incoming state names. Per transition, the information resembles the output of the standard `summary.survfit` function in the **survival** package. Each observed transition time, of whatever type, and each censoring time generates one row. Hence, the same time points appear in every component, even if a time point corresponds to another transition. Unlike the `summary.survfit` function, there is no `times` argument to select specific time points. We obtain the estimates for the transition from SI to AIDS/SI at some arbitrary time points via

```
Summ.Prob.etm <- summary(Prob.etm, ci.fun="log")
Summ.Prob.etm[["SI AIDS/SI"]][seq(100,400,by=100),]
```

yielding

	P	time	var	lower	upper	n.risk	n.event
1.990	0.0000	1.99	0.00000	NaN	NaN	12	0
3.647	0.1655	3.65	0.00803	0.0573	0.478	24	0
5.478	0.2250	5.48	0.01073	0.0912	0.555	32	0
6.829	0.1425	6.83	0.00460	0.0561	0.362	37	0

The `summary.etm` function also gives the probabilities to remain in a state. For example, the probability to remain in the initial state is obtained via

---

[7]In order to avoid confusion as to which columns are chosen, it is better not to have all three column names—entry, exit and time—in the same data set (as was the case in Table 3.2).

[8]The **from** and **to** columns need to be factors that include all the defined states as levels.

`Summ.Prob.etm[["HIV HIV"]]`. If the output of the `summary.etm` function is not assigned to an object, it directly returns its output to the output window. By default this is done for six time points[9], but if the argument `all` is set to `TRUE` it is done for all time points.

The estimate of the variance is based on the Greenwood formula. The scale at which the confidence intervals are computed is specified via the `ci.fun`. The default is the linear scale. Other options are `"cloglog"` for the complementary log-log scale as defined in (1.21) and (1.22) on Page 35. The complementary log-log scale in (1.23) is specified via `"log-log"`. The log scale in (1.23) is specified via `"log"`; the other log scale is not supported. The default value of the `level` argument is 0.95.

Summarizing results via ***trprob.etm*** *and* ***trcov.etm***

If we want to summarize the Aalen-Johansen estimate for a transition that does not have a direct path, we use the `trprob.etm` function. The required arguments are the estimate as obtained via the `etm` function and the transition of interest. The output of `trprob.etm` is a named vector. The values are the estimates and the names are the corresponding time points. By default, it gives the transition probability at all time points with an observed transition, of whatever type, and at all time points with an observed censoring. Time points can be chosen via the optional `timepoints` argument. As example, we compute the transition probabilities from HIV to death at the same time points as above.

```
Prob.hiv.death <- trprob(Prob.etm, tr.choice=c("HIV death"))
Prob.hiv.death[seq(100,400,by=100)]
```

gives

```
    1.9903052703628 3.64691649555084        5.4784 6.82859274469547
        0.008044077      0.037275969   0.135194871      0.246647691
```

For a more extensive summary with confidence intervals you are advised to combine time and estimates into a data frame, e.g. via

```
Prob.hiv.death <- data.frame(
    time=as.numeric(names(Prob.hiv.death)), prob=Prob.hiv.death)
```

Confidence intervals are based on the variance estimate $\widehat{\mathrm{var}}\{\widehat{P_{gh}}(s,t)\}$ as obtained via the `trcov.etm` function. For example, for the transition from HIV to death we can add confidence intervals on the log scale as in (1.20) via

```
tmp <- trcov(Prob.etm, tr.choice=c("HIV death"))
Prob.hiv.death$lower.ci <- pmax(0,1-(1-Prob.hiv.death$prob)*
            exp(qnorm(0.975)*sqrt(tmp)/(1-Prob.hiv.death$prob)))
Prob.hiv.death$upper.ci <- 1-(1-Prob.hiv.death$prob)*
            exp(-qnorm(0.975)*sqrt(tmp)/(1-Prob.hiv.death$prob))
```

---

[9]The quantiles 0, 0.25, 0.5, 0.75, 0.9, and 1.

Note that this scale is currently not supplied by the `summary.etm` function.

We can also combine transitions. Since the times at which the estimates are computed are the same for all transitions, it is easy to combine estimates. The estimated transition probability from HIV to either of the states AIDS or AIDS/SI as shown in Figure 3.8 can be computed via

```
Prob.hiv.aids <- trprob(Prob.etm, "HIV AIDS") +
                              trprob(Prob.etm, "HIV AIDS/SI")
```

The file `ExampleCode.R` on the book's website shows how the confidence intervals can be computed for this combined end point. For this we also need an estimate of the covariance $\widehat{\text{covar}}\{\widehat{P}_{gh}(s,t), \widehat{P}_{g'h'}(s,t)\}$, which is also obtained via the `trcov.etm` function.

Plotting the results

The `etm` package has a `plot.etm` function that is easy to use and suffices in many situations. The `tr.choice` argument allows for specifying the transitions of interest as a character vector; transitions that do not have a direct path can be chosen as well. Plots are always drawn in overlaid display format.

```
plot(Prob.etm , tr.choice=c("HIV death"), conf.int=TRUE,
                                          ci.fun="log")
```

If we do not specify `tr.choice` then the probabilities are plotted for all transitions that have a direct path, as in Figure 3.5. A similar function exists to plot the cumulative transition hazards based on the `mvna` output.

If we want to have more flexibility, we can first create a data frame with all estimates, after which we use any type of `plot` function. The code that created the Figures 3.4 to 3.9 is given in the file `ExampleCode.R`.

3.7.2   The `msSurv` package

Specify allowed transitions

The allowed transitions are specified via a `graphNEL` object, which is defined in the `graph` package. Before being able to load the `msSurv` package, you first need to install the `graph` package from the bioconductor repository (see the code in the file `ExampleCode.R` on the book's website). Our 5-state model can be specified via

```
Nodes <- c("HIV","AIDS","SI","AIDS/SI","death")
Edges <- list("HIV" = list(edges=c("AIDS","SI")),
              "AIDS" = list(edges=c("AIDS/SI","death")),
              "SI" = list(edges=c("AIDS/SI")),
              "AIDS/SI" = list(edges=c("death")),
              "death" = list(edges=NULL))
ms.Diag <- new("graphNEL", nodes=Nodes, edgeL=Edges,
                                        edgemode="directed")
```

First we define the states. The allowed direct transitions are specified in a named list. Each component of the list refers to one state and is itself a list that specifies the states that can be reached next.

Create data set

msSurv does not contain a function to create the data set in the required transition-based format. One option is to use the etmprep function from the etm package and change column names and state values in the resulting data set (code shown in ExampleCode.R). We call the resulting data set aidssi.msSurv.

The computations

Both the Nelson-Aalen and the Aalen-Johansen estimate are computed via the msSurv function. The only required arguments are the data and the graphNEL object. The column names are required to be as specified in Table 3.5, i.e. **id**, **start.stage**, **end.stage**, **start** and **stop**. For a Markov renewal process without left truncation, the **start** column is not needed. The values of the states can be character or numeric; censored observations need to have the value 0.

The estimates in Section 3.4.2 were computed via

```
Prob.msSurv <- msSurv(aidssi.msSurv, ms.Diag, LT=TRUE)
```

If aidssi.msSurv has more columns, we need to select the five mentioned above, e.g. aidssi.msSurv Since we have late entry, we need to set LT to TRUE.

Summarizing results

The summary function sends summary information to the console window but the result cannot be stored in an object. It gives the transition probabilities for the transitions that have a direct path, the state occupation probabilities, as well as the entry and exit time distributions. We can leave each of them out by setting the arguments stateocc, trans.pr and dist to FALSE. By default results are shown at five time points[10], but if the argument all is set to TRUE estimates are shown for all time points. We can also choose specific time points at which we want to have the information by using the times argument. The scale at which the confidence intervals are computed is specified via the ci.fun argument; the default is the linear scale. The level argument is 0.95 by default.

If we want to have more control, we use another approach. The output of msSurv is an S4 class. An S4 class has slots, and it is easy to obtain the numeric results from these slots. The most important slots are i) et for the transition times, ii) I.dA for the matrices $\mathbf{I} + \widehat{d\Lambda}(u)$ that are the components

---

[10]The quartiles 0, 0.25, 0.5, 0.75, and 1.

of the Aalen-Johansen estimate (3.9); note that the off-diagonal elements are the increments of the Nelson-Aalen estimate, iii) `AJs` and `cov.AJs` for the Aalen-Johansen estimate and the estimate of the variance $\widehat{\mathrm{var}}\{\widehat{P_{gh}}(s,t)\}$, iv) `ps` and `var.sop` for the estimated state occupation probabilities and their variances, v) `Fsub` and `Fsub.var` for the estimates of the state entry distributions and their variances, vi) `Gsub` and `Gsub.var` for the estimates of the state exit distributions and their variances. All variance estimates are based on the Greenwood formula.

For example, estimates of all transition probabilities from the time origin $s = 0$ and their variances can be obtained via

```
trProb.est <- AJs(Prob.msSurv)
trProb.var <- cov.AJs(Prob.msSurv)
```

Both are three-dimensional arrays. The first two dimensions specify the transitions, the third dimension contains the estimates. There is an estimate at each observed transition time, of whatever type, and at each censoring time. For example, a data frame with the estimates for the transition from HIV to death, together with confidence intervals on the log scale (1.20), can be obtained via

```
Prob.hiv.death <- data.frame(time=et(Prob.msSurv),
                      prob=trProb.est[1,5,],
                  var=trProb.var["HIV death","HIV death",])
Prob.hiv.death$lower.ci <- pmax(0,1-(1-Prob.hiv.death$prob)*
                                  exp(qnorm(0.975)*
          sqrt(Prob.hiv.death$var)/(1-Prob.hiv.death$prob)))
Prob.hiv.death$upper.ci <- 1-(1-Prob.hiv.death$prob)*
                                  exp(-qnorm(0.975)*
          sqrt(Prob.hiv.death$var)/(1-Prob.hiv.death$prob))
```

Note that array elements start at 1, not at 0. Therefore, we need to write `trProb.est[1,5,]` to select the transitions out of state 0, HIV.

If we want to estimate the transition probabilities starting from a later time point, for example from 4 years, we compute the Aalen-Johansen estimator (3.9) ourselves by taking a product of matrices that are contained in the `I.dA` slot:

```
## idx gives the indices of the event times after 4 years
idx <- which(4 <= et(Prob.msSurv))
trProb.est4 <- array(0,dim=c(5,5,length(idx)))
trProb.est4[ , ,1] <- I.dA(Prob.msSurv)[ , ,idx[1]]
for (i in 2:length(idx)) trProb.est4[ , ,i] <-
        trProb.est4[ , ,i-1] %*% I.dA(Prob.msSurv)[ , ,idx[i]]
```

We can also combine transitions. For example, a data frame with the estimated transition probability from HIV to either of the states AIDS or AIDS/SI, as shown in Figure 3.8, is obtained via

```
Prob.1to24 <- AJs(Prob.msSurv)[1,2,] + AJs(Prob.msSurv)[1,4,]
Prob.1to24 <- data.frame(time=et(Prob.msSurv), prob=Prob.1to24)
```

The file `ExampleCode.R` shows how the confidence intervals can be computed for the combined end point. For this we also need an estimate of the covariance $\widehat{\text{covar}}\{\widehat{P}_{gh}(s,t), \widehat{P}_{g'h'}(s,t)\}$ between both estimators, which is also provided by the `cov.AJs` slot.

For a fixed horizon prediction we again compute the Aalen-Johansen estimator by taking a product of matrices that are contained in the `I.dA` slot. We need to change the direction of matrix multiplication, because the first time variable s is the one that varies. The computations that led to Figure 3.10 are

```
idx <- which(et(Prob.msSurv)≥2 & et(Prob.msSurv) ≤10)
n.tm <- length(idx)
FixedHor10 <- array(0,dim=c(5,5,n.tm))
FixedHor10[,,n.tm] <- I.dA(Prob.msSurv)[,,idx[n.tm]]
for (i in (n.tm-1):1) FixedHor10[,,i] <-
                I.dA(Prob.msSurv)[,,idx[i]]%*%FixedHor10[,,i+1]
```

The package also contains the function `Pst`, which estimates the transition probability between two specific time points, as well as the functions `SOPt` and `EntryExit` that estimate the state occupation probability and state entry/exit distributions at one specific time point. The variance of the estimate is included by setting the `covar` argument to `TRUE`. For example, the matrix of transition probabilities between $s = 4$ and $t = 10$ is obtained via

```
Pst(Prob.msSurv, s=4, t=10)
```

which yields

```
Estimate of P(4, 10)
          cols
          HIV    AIDS      SI AIDS/SI   death
  HIV     0.4175 0.0880 0.1224  0.0344 0.3377
  AIDS    0.0000 0.0368 0.0000  0.0042 0.9589
  SI      0.0000 0.0000 0.1506  0.0668 0.7826
  AIDS/SI 0.0000 0.0000 0.0000  0.0153 0.9847
  death   0.0000 0.0000 0.0000  0.0000 1.0000
```

Plotting the results

The `msSurv` package has its own function for plotting results; plots are based on the `lattice` package. For example, all state occupation probabilities can be plotted via

```
plot(Prob.msSurv, plot.type="stateocc")
```

Often we want to have more control. We can make plots by selecting the relevant components from the slots of the `msSurv` output. The code that created the Figures 3.4 to 3.9 can be found in the file `ExampleCode.R`.

3.7.3 The `mstate` package

Specify allowed transitions

The elements in the matrix that correspond to the allowed direct transitions are numbered, starting at 1. The other transitions have the value NA. We can create the transition matrix with the function `transMat` in `mstate`. Its first argument is a list, which consists of vectors that specify the states to where direct transitions are possible. Our 5-state model can be defined via

```
trans.mst <- transMat(
        x = list(c(2, 3), c(4, 5), c(4), c(5), c()),
        names = c("HIV", "AIDS", "SI", "AIDS/SI", "death"))
```

which results in the following matrix

```
          to
from      HIV AIDS SI AIDS/SI death
  HIV      NA    1  2      NA    NA
  AIDS     NA   NA NA       3     4
  SI       NA   NA NA       5    NA
  AIDS/SI  NA   NA NA      NA     6
  death    NA   NA NA      NA    NA
```

For clarity we have given names to the rows and columns that correspond to the states, but this is not required. There are special functions `trans.comprisk` and `trans.illdeath` to define competing risks models and illness-death models (see Section 5.7.1 for an example of the use of `trans.comprisk`). The functions number the transitions row-wise. If we want another numbering we have to create the matrix ourselves.

Create data set

The `mstate` package requires the data to be in stacked long format. It can be created from a data set in wide state-ordered format using the `msprep` function. Its arguments resemble the ones in `crprep`, which was explained in Section 2.9.1.2. Similar to `crprep`, we can specify the required information either by giving the actual data or by giving the names of the columns that contain this information. We describe the latter specification.

`msprep` has as required arguments 1) `time`: a vector with the names of the columns that specify the transition (or censoring) times, one for every possible state, and given in the same order as in the transition matrix; 2) `status`: a vector of the same length as in 1) that has the names of the corresponding status columns; in each column, the value should be 1 if the state was reached and 0 if not; 3) `data`: the name of the data set[11] 4) `trans`: the matrix that defines the allowed transitions.

The initial state is one of the states in the model and should be included

---

[11]This argument is not used if we give the actual data.

in the vectors of column names in the `time` and `status` arguments. If the data set does not contain these columns, we can use `NA` as a column name. Before explaining the optional arguments, we first provide the code:

```
aidssi.mst <- msprep(
  time=c(NA,"aids.time","si.time","siaids.time","death.time"),
  status=c(NA,"aids.stat","si.stat","siaids.stat","death.stat"),
  data=aidssi2, trans=trans.mst,
 start=list(time=aidssi2$entry.time,state=rep(1,nrow(aidssi2))))
```

The arguments `start`, `id` and `keep` serve similar purposes as in the `crprep` function. Late entry is specified via the `start` argument. Contrary to `crprep`, this argument does not accept column names; we have to provide the values of the entry times and the values of the initial states via a list structure with components named `time` and `state`. All individuals in our data set started in state HIV. The `id` argument can be used to keep the original values of the person indentifiers. Other variables can be copied to the data set via the `keep` argument.

The result of `msprep` is a data frame in stacked format with the transition matrix as attribute[12]. The multi-state information is given in columns named **from**, **to**, **trans**, **Tstart**, **Tstop**, **time** and **status**. The columns **Tstart** and **Tstop** give the time of entry into and exit from the state value in **from**. There is a row for every possible state that can be reached from **from**; the incoming state is given in **to**. All states have numeric values, starting at 1. The corresponding transition number, as defined in the transition matrix, is in **trans**. For the four example individuals in Table 3.1, the result is shown in Table 4.5. For the computations, the names and ordering of the columns in the stacked data set do not matter.

The computations

Computations go in three steps. We start with computing the Nelson-Aalen estimates via a proportional hazards model without covariables but with transition as stratum variable. The stacked format allows us to compute them for all direct transitions in one go. We use[13]

```
NA.surv <- coxph(Surv(Tstart,Tstop,status)~strata(trans),
                                        data=aidssi.mst)
```

The next step is to apply the `msfit` function, which restructures the Nelson-Aalen estimates in another format. This intermediate step is included because `msfit` also serves to compute the estimate of the cumulative transition hazard based on a regression model, for an individual with a specific covariable combination (see Section 5.7.1). We use

---

[12]It is an object of class *msdata*.

[13]If there are ties in the data, we need to specify `ties="breslow"` in order to obtain the Aalen-Johansen estimator of the transition probability.

```
NA.mst <- msfit(NA.mst, vartype="greenwood", trans=trans.mst)
```

Note that the default is the Aalen estimator of the variance[14]. The output has a list structure. The first component, named `Haz`, is a data frame with columns **time**, **Haz** (the estimates) and **trans** (the transitions that the estimates refer to). The cumulative hazard estimates for all transitions are contained in a single column. The second component, named `varHaz`, contains the variances and covariances of the estimated cumulative hazards. It is a data frame with columns `time`, `varHaz`, `trans1` and `trans2`. The combination of values in `trans1` and `trans2` determines what the value in `varHaz` estimates: the rows in which they have the same value give the estimated variances for the transitions. If `trans1` and `trans2` differ, they give the covariances for two different transitions $\widehat{\text{covar}}\{\widehat{\Lambda_{gh}}(t), \widehat{\Lambda_{g'h'}}(t)\}$.

The final step is to compute the transition probabilities via the `probtrans` function. The `probtrans` function has two required arguments. The first is the output of the `msfit` function. The second is the time point from which we want the computations in case of fixed history prediction. In order to compute all transition probabilities from the time origin, we write

```
Prob.mst <- probtrans(NA.mst, predt=0, method="greenwood")
```

The transition probabilities from $s = 4$ are obtained by specifying `predt=4`. By default, standard errors are stored in the output, but if we also want the covariances we need to specify `covariance=TRUE`.

In case of fixed horizon prediction, we change the value of the `direction` argument in `probtrans` to `"fixedhorizon"`. Now the value in `predt` defines the horizon t and we compute $P_{gh}(s,t)$ for varying s. To obtain the prediction at the fixed horizon ten years after HIV infection (Figure 3.10), we use

```
Prob.mst.R <- probtrans(NA.mst, predt=10,
                              direction="fixedhorizon")
```

Summarizing results

If we apply the **summary** function to the `probtrans` output, estimates for all transitions are shown in the output console window. It only shows the estimates at the first and last six time points, unless the argument `complete` is set to `TRUE`. Transition probabilities from one specific state are obtained using the `from` argument. Since estimates cannot be assigned to an R object, the function is not very useful.

We better directly use the information as stored in the `probtrans` output. It has a list structure with one component per outgoing state. Each component is a data frame with the estimated transition probabilites from that state. It has columns with names `time`, `pstate1` etc. for the estimates and `se1` etc. for the standard errors. Hence, the same time points appear in every component,

---

[14]It is also possible to leave out the variance estimates by specifying `variance=FALSE`.

also time points that correspond to transitions from other states. Confidence intervals are not supplied, we need to compute them ourselves. For example, a data frame with the estimates and confidence intervals, on the log scale (1.19), for the transition from HIV to death can be obtained via

```
Prob.hiv.death <- data.frame(time=Prob.mst[[1]]$time,
            prob=Prob.mst[[1]]$pstate5, se=Prob.mst[[1]]$se5)
Prob.hiv.death$lower.ci <- pmax(0,1-(1-Prob.hiv.death$prob)*
                           exp(qnorm(0.975)*
            Prob.hiv.death$se/(1-Prob.hiv.death$prob)))
Prob.hiv.death$upper.ci <- 1-(1-Prob.hiv.death$prob)*
                           exp(-qnorm(0.975)*
            Prob.hiv.death$se/(1-Prob.hiv.death$prob))
```

Each component stores estimates for all transition times, also if they are for a transition from another outgoing state, as well as for all censoring times. Therefore, it is easy to combine information from different transitions in one data frame. For example, the estimate of the transition probability from HIV to either of the states AIDS or AIDS/SI as shown in Figure 3.8 is computed via

```
Prob.hiv.aids <- data.frame(time=Prob.mst[[1]]$time,
            P=Prob.mst[[1]]$pstate2+Prob.mst[[1]]$pstate4)
```

The file `ExampleCode.R` on the book's website shows how the confidence intervals can be computed for the combined end point.

Plotting the results

The `mstate` package has a `plot.probtrans` function that is easy to use and suffices for many situations. If we want to plot transition probabilities from one specific state only, we use the argument `from`. Another argument is `type`, which allows us to choose between the display formats that were described on Page 66. For example, all transition probabilities out of the HIV state, the state occupation probabilities in Figure 3.7, can be plotted via

```
plot(Prob.mst, type="single")
```

Note that `from=1` is the default. If these functions do not suffice we can always make plots by selecting the relevant components from the `probtrans` output. The code that created the Figures 3.4 to 3.9 is given in `ExampleCode.R`.

3.8   Computer practicals

We look beyond relapse and also quantify the transition hazard and transition probability from relapse to death. We use a multi-state model with three states, 1: Transplant (T), 2: Relapse (R), and 3: Death (D). There are three possible transitions: 1: T → R, 2: R → D and 3: T → D. You can use either of the packages `etm`, `msSurv` and `mstate`.

1. **Define the structure** Make a directed graph of the multi-state model. Indicate the state numbers and names as well as the transition numbers.

2. **Create the stacked data set** What is the format of the `ebmt1` data set? Transform it into a format that can be used for estimation of the transition probabilities.

   Compare the data of the first two patients with those in the original wide format and see whether this makes sense to you.

3. **Estimation of cumulative hazard** Compute the cumulative hazard function for all three transitions, using a clock-forward approach. Plot them in one single figure in overlaid display format. If an individual is still free of relapse, which of the events is more likely to happen, relapse or death? What is the effect of relapse on the mortality rate?

   Compare the estimate for the transition from relapse to death with the one that is computed based on a Cox model without covariables. Add this estimate to the plot.

4. **Estimation of transition probabilities** Estimate the fixed history transition probabilities for all three transitions from the time origin onwards. Give a numeric summary of the state prevalence at 5 years after transplant. Compute the estimates as well as the 95% confidence intervals on the linear scale as defined in (1.18) on Page 34.

5. **Creation of informative plots** Make two different plots, without confidence intervals:

   1. All three state occupation probabilities in stacked format.
   2. Transition probabilities for the three transitions T → R, R → D and T → D, in overlaid format.

   Answer the following questions:

   - What is the relation between the three curves in the first figure.
   - Why can the curves in the second figure add up to a number larger than one?
   - Which of the curves in the second figure can also decrease over time? Why?
   - Why is the transition probability much higher from transplantation to death than from transplantation to relapse, whereas this is not seen for the cumulative hazards?

5. **Time from transplantation to death** Compare the estimated distribution of time from transplantation to death using the classical Kaplan-Meier and using the multi-state Aalen-Johansen estimator. Also plot and compare the 95% confidence intervals.

4

Regression; Cause-Specific/Transition Hazard

4.1 Introduction

In the previous chapters, we quantified the transition and state occupation probabilities for the population as a whole. Often, we also want to know whether and how these depend on characteristics that vary within the population. If we are interested in a single categorical characteristic like gender or CCR5 genotype, we can estimate them separately for each value. And they can be compared via a nonparametric test as described in Sections 1.11.5 and 2.6. Beyond this situation, we need to make further assumptions and specify some type of regression model in which effects are quantified through parameters.

The most popular approach is the proportional hazards model, in which effects are quantified via parameters, which are assumed constant over follow-up time. In this chapter, we concentrate on models that assume proportional cause-specific hazards, which immediately generalize to transition hazards in the multi-state setting. In Chapter 5, we look at some ways to quantify effects on the cumulative scale. One of them has a similar structure: the proportional subdistribution hazards model.

In Section 4.2, the basic structure of the proportional cause-specific hazards model is adressed. Estimation is completely standard. We are fitting a Cox proportional hazards model; only the interpretation is different. We can fit one model per end point or transition, but a more powerful analysis is to combine all competing events or transitions into one analysis. The main purpose of this chapter is to describe the data format that is needed for such a combined analysis and to explain the extra flexibility that is gained. The main difficulty is in defining the proper contrasts and the interpretation of the parameter estimates. In Section 4.3 we describe how the combined analysis is performed in the competing risks setting by means of the simplest example of a dichotomous covariable and two types of end points. In Section 4.4 we explain why this approach gives valid estimates. This section is more technical; its contents is not used in the sequel and can be skipped if you are more interested in the application. In Section 4.5 the ideas are extended to the multi-state setting, again by means of an example. In Section 4.6 we give a detailed description of the choice of contrasts and their interpretation via an example on the effect of combined HIV and HCV infection on progression to four different causes of death.

Since everything boils down to fitting standard Cox models, analyses can be performed in any program for survival analysis. Throughout this chapter, we use R code as example. Users of other programs can adapt the basic ideas to their setting.

We denote the covariables of subject i by $\mathbf{Z}_i$. We make the assumption that the late entry and right censoring mechanisms are non-informative for what happens with respect to progression to the subsequent state, but this time we only require it to hold conditionally on the covariables in the model.

4.2 Regression on cause-specific hazard: basic structure

In a proportional cause-specific hazards model, the effect of the covariables on the cause-specific hazard for cause k is described via

$$\lambda_k(t \mid \mathbf{Z}_i) = \lambda_{k,0}(t) \exp(\boldsymbol{\beta}_k^\top \mathbf{Z}_i). \tag{4.1}$$

The only difference with the Cox proportional hazards model in the classical setting (see (1.27) on Page 37) is that now everything refers to a specific type of end point via the subscript k. The parameters $\boldsymbol{\beta}_k$ quantify the effect of the covariables $\mathbf{Z}_i$ on the progression rate to cause k and $\lambda_{k,0}(t)$ is the baseline cause-specific hazard for cause k.

In Section 2.3 it was explained that the cause-specific hazard can be estimated by removing individuals from the risk set when they experience a competing event. As a consequence, the estimation procedure is the same as in the classical setting with only one type of end point. When fitting model (4.1), we can use all the techniques that are used when fitting a standard Cox proportional hazards model (see Sections 1.8.4 and 1.8.5). The difference is in the interpretation: we quantify effects on the cause-specific hazard, not on the marginal hazard. Only if the censoring due to the competing risks is non-informative conditionally on the covariables in the model, then the estimates can also be interpreted as effects on the marginal hazard. Since a different quantity is estimated, we call it a proportional cause-specific hazards model and not a Cox model. Using this name also emphasizes the distinction with the proportional subdistribution hazards model, often called the Fine and Gray model (Section 5.3).

We use the `aidssi` data set as example. On Page 54 we quantified the effect of the CCR5-Δ32 deletion on progression to the combined SI/AIDS end point via a Cox model. We observed that individuals with the deletion had a smaller progression rate. In this section we analyse this effect separately for SI switch and AIDS as first event. A schematic representation of our model is given in Figure 4.1. We choose `WW` as the reference category. The baseline hazards $\lambda_{1,0}$ and $\lambda_{2,0}$ describe the AIDS-specific and SI-specific hazards for the reference group. For the individuals with the deletion, these hazards are multiplied by a

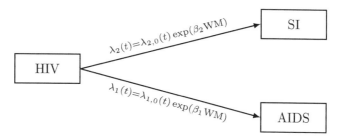

FIGURE 4.1
Schematic representation of the effect of the CCR5-Δ32 deletion on each of
the competing events.

factor $\exp(\beta_1)$ and $\exp(\beta_2)$ respectively. In the first five columns of Table 4.1
we repeat the information from the individuals in rows 14, 3, 15 and 8 (see
Table 1.3 on Page 51).

TABLE 4.1
Four example individuals from `aidssi` data set

patnr	time	status	cause	ccr5	status1	status2
14	5.05	0	event-free	WW	0	0
3	2.23	1	AIDS	WW	1	0
15	10.20	1	AIDS	WM	1	0
8	8.61	2	SI	WW	0	1

If we quantify the effect of CCR5 on the AIDS-specific hazard, only the
individuals that were observed to develop AIDS before an SI switch have an
event. These are the individuals that have the value 1 in the **status** column
or the value `AIDS` in the **cause** column. All other individuals are treated as
right censored. If we use the **status** column we can write

```
coxph(Surv(time, status==1) ~ ccr5, data = aidssi)
```

`status==1` is a logical statement with outcomes `FALSE` or `TRUE`, which are
interpreted as 0 and 1. We added these values as extra column **status1** to
Table 4.1. We obtain

```
          coef exp(coef) se(coef)      z      p
ccr5WM  -1.24     0.291    0.307  -4.02 5.7e-05


Likelihood ratio test=22  on 1 df, p=2.76e-06   n= 324,
                                  number of events= 113
   (5 observations deleted due to missingness)
```

For the switch to SI phenotype as the first event, we only need to redefine the
event in the **status** variable as being equal to 2, which results in the values
in the column **status2**. Using

```
coxph(Surv(time, status==2) ~ ccr5, data = aidssi)
```

we obtain

```
          coef exp(coef) se(coef)      z      p
ccr5WM -0.254     0.776    0.238 -1.07   0.29

Likelihood ratio test=1.19  on 1 df, p=0.275  n= 324,
                                number of events= 107
   (5 observations deleted due to missingness)
```

We observe that individuals with the deletion have a slower progression rate to the combined AIDS/SI end point mainly because of their lower AIDS-specific hazard. The relative hazard $\exp(\beta_{AIDS}) = 0.291$ is significantly different from 1. The estimated SI-specific hazard for individuals with the deletion is only slightly lower than the hazard for those without the deletion, but the relative hazard $\exp(\beta_{SI}) = 0.776$ is not significantly different from one.

We fitted a separate model for each end point. This resembles a stratified regression analysis. A stratified analysis is performed if the effect of covariables is quantified separately for each value of some categorical variable such as gender. The main reason to perform a stratified analysis is simplicity; the parameters are easy to interpret. However, exactly the same results are obtained by fitting one regression model that includes gender as extra covariable and that allows the effect of all other covariables to be modified by gender via interaction terms. Using one single model with interaction terms has several advantages. We can *test* whether the effect of the covariables differs by gender. And if we want to *assume* the effect of a covariable to be the same for both genders, we can remove the interaction term from the model. This increases power if the assumption is correct.

Similarly, in the above competing risks analyses per end point, we cannot test the hypothesis whether the effect of the deletion is the same for both end points, i.e. whether $\beta_{AIDS} = \beta_{SI}$. And we cannot perform an analysis in which β_{AIDS} and β_{SI} are assumed to be equal. Also, we cannot test whether hazards for different causes are proportional or fit models in which we assume baseline cause-specific hazards to be proportional. For this, we need to create an augmented data set using a duplication method [69]. In the next section we explain the structure of such a data set.

4.3   Combined analysis and type-specific covariables

The above two analyses per end point used the same time and covariable information. Only the definition of the event via the `status` variable was different. If we want to perform the analysis for both end points at once, we stack the data as used in each separate analysis.

In Table 4.2 we show the data of the four example individuals from Table 4.1 in the stacked format. The **time** and **ccr5** variables from the original data set are duplicated. The data has an extra column **failcode**, denoting which of the two separate analyses the information in that row comes from. Hence, per individual one row has the value AIDS and one row has the value SI. Unlike **ccr5**, it is not a characteristic of the individual. Every individual is at risk to progress to either of the two end points and thus has both values of **failcode**. The **status** variable has the value 1 if the values in **cause** and **failcode** coincide, and 0 otherwise.

TABLE 4.2
Four example individuals in the stacked long format

patnr	time	status	cause	failcode	ccr5
14	5.05	0	event-free	AIDS	WW
14	5.05	0	event-free	SI	WW
3	2.23	1	AIDS	AIDS	WW
3	2.23	0	AIDS	SI	WW
15	10.20	1	AIDS	AIDS	WM
15	10.20	0	AIDS	SI	WM
8	8.61	0	SI	AIDS	WW
8	8.61	1	SI	SI	WW

If there are K competing events, each individual has K rows in the stacked format.

The original data set is used for the separate analyses; if we want to combine the end points into one analysis we enlarge the data set. This is different from a normal stratified analysis. If we want to stratify the analysis by the values of some variable, we start with one data set that contains information from all individuals and split the data.

4.3.1 Same results in one analysis

If we perform the analysis per end point, each analysis yields its own estimates of the baseline hazard and of the effect of the deletion. In the combined analysis, we estimate a separate baseline hazard per end point by including the type of end point as stratum variable in the model. The separate effect of the CCR5-Δ32 deletion per end point can be modeled in several ways. The most straightforward, but not the most elegant way is by including an interaction between **ccr5** and **failcode**. If we call the stacked data set **aidssi.stack**, we use[1]

```
coxph(Surv(time, status) ~ ccr5 * strata(failcode),
                                    data = aidssi.stack)
```

---

[1] In R, the asterisk in the regression formula is used to denote both the main effects and their interaction.

which yields the following output[2]

```
                       coef exp(coef) se(coef)     z       p
ccr5WM               -1.236     0.291    0.307 -4.02 5.7e-05
ccr5WM:strata(failcode)f 0.982  2.669    0.389  2.53 1.2e-02


Likelihood ratio test=23.2  on 2 df, p=9.29e-06  n= 648,
                                number of events= 220
    (10 observations deleted due to missingness)
```

Since `failcode` is a stratum variable, it does not have a main effect estimate. The value -1.236 is, as before, the effect of the deletion on the AIDS-specific hazard. The value 0.982 is different from the earlier analyses. It represents the *additional* effect of the deletion on the SI-specific hazard. The effect -0.254 that we found in the separate analysis with SI as the end point can also be reproduced. It is the effect on AIDS plus the additional effect that is represented by the interaction term: $-1.236 + 0.982 = -0.254$ (or equivalently the product of 0.291 and 2.669 is equal to 0.776 on the scale of the hazard). Note that the value of the likelihood ratio test statistic is the sum of the two values from the separate analyses.

We see the first advantage of the use of the stacked data format. We can test whether the effect of the CCR5-Δ32 deletion is the same for the AIDS-specific and the SI-specific hazard via the interaction term. Since it is significant with $p = 0.012$, we conclude that the effect of the CCR5-Δ32 deletion on the cause-specific hazards is not equal.

Instead of including an interaction term, we can also create a compound variable that combines information on CCR5 and end point. We create a categorical variable with three levels: the baseline WW level and two levels for the deletion in order to allow the effect of WM to depend on type of end point. This is the column **ccr.comb** in Table 4.3. Contrary to the standard regression setting we have three instead of four levels, because the baseline hazards are estimated nonparametrically.

We fit a model with this new variable via

```
fit.stacked <- coxph(Surv(time, status) ~ ccr.comb +
                      strata(failcode), data = aidssi.stack)
```

We obtain exactly the same parameter estimates, standard errors and resulting p-values as in the analyses per end point:

```
                  coef exp(coef) se(coef)     z       p
ccr.combWM.AIDS -1.236     0.291    0.307 -4.02 5.7e-05
ccr.combWM.SI   -0.254     0.776    0.238 -1.07 2.9e-01
```

In Section 4.4.1 we explain why results are equal.

A stratified proportional hazards model is not the same as a stratified analysis. A stratified analysis is performed when models are fitted separately

---

[2]We have abbreviated the name of the second row in the output table.

TABLE 4.3

Four example individuals in the stacked long format with compound and type-specific variables

patnr	time	status	failcode	ccr5	ccr.comb	ccrAIDS	ccrSI
14	5.05	0	AIDS	WW	WW	0	0
14	5.05	0	SI	WW	WW	0	0
3	2.23	1	AIDS	WW	WW	0	0
3	2.23	0	SI	WW	WW	0	0
15	10.20	1	AIDS	WM	WM.AIDS	1	0
15	10.20	0	SI	WM	WM.SI	0	1
8	8.61	0	AIDS	WW	WW	0	0
8	8.61	1	SI	WW	WW	0	0

for each value of some categorical variable. A stratified proportional hazards model is a single proportional hazards model in which a separate baseline hazard is estimated for each value of a categorical variable. If we include an interaction between the stratum variable and every other variable in the model, all parameters are stratum-specific. Fitting a stratified proportional hazards model is the same as fitting a separate proportional hazards model for each value of the stratum variable. This is in the same spirit as the equivalence between a stratified analysis and a model that includes an interaction between the categorical variable and all other variables (see Page 146).

There has been some controversy surrounding the calculation of the standard error in the combined analysis. A sandwich-type robust estimator of the standard error was suggested in order to correct for the fact that individuals are replicated in the stacked data set [69]. If we use a robust estimate via

```
coxph(Surv(time, status) ~ ccr.comb + strata(failcode)
                    + cluster(patnr), data = aidssi.stack)
```

we observe that the standard errors and p-values are no longer equal to the ones from the separate analyses, although the difference is small:

	coef	se(coef)	p	robust se	robust p
ccr.combWM.AIDS	-1.236	0.307	0.00005	0.296	0.00003
ccr.combWM.SI	-0.254	0.238	0.28555	0.233	0.27480

Only the non-robust standard errors replicate the results from the separate analyses. The reason is that individuals can experience one event at most (see Section 4.4.1).

4.3.2 Type-specific covariables

Since we cannot compute on text representations, statistical programs first transform the categorical variable **ccr.comb** into two dummy variables that represent the non-reference values `WM.AIDS` and `WM.SI`. They are given in the columns **ccrAIDS** and **ccrSI** in Table 4.3. The variable **ccrAIDS** has the value 1 when neither the genotype is the reference category nor the event type in **failcode** has the value `AIDS`, and it has the value 0 otherwise (see person 15); similarly for **ccrSI** and `SI`. The same parameter estimates and p-values as above are obtained if we directly use the two dummy variables instead of **ccr.comb**:

```
coxph(Surv(time, status) ~ ccrAIDS + ccrSI + strata(failcode),
                                          data = aidssi.stack)
```

The variables **ccrSI** and **ccrAIDS** are called type-specific covariables [6, p.478].

The basic idea behind the use of type-specific covariables is that, instead of using the covariables $\mathbf{Z}_i$ in the original data set and specifying

$$\lambda_k(t \mid \mathbf{Z}_i) = \lambda_{k,0}(t) \, \exp(\boldsymbol{\beta}_k^\top \mathbf{Z}_i) \,,$$

we can equivalently specify

$$\lambda_k(t \mid \mathbf{Z}_i) = \lambda_{k,0}(t) \, \exp(\boldsymbol{\beta}^\top \mathbf{Z}_{k,i}) \,.$$

The type-specific covariable $\mathbf{Z}_{k,i}$ equals $\mathbf{Z}_i$ for cause k, and has value 0 otherwise. The parameters $\boldsymbol{\beta}_k$ that are modeled for each separate analysis are replaced by one set of parameters $\boldsymbol{\beta}$ that model the effect of all type-specific covariables. In the CCR5 example we have one variable, $Z_i = \text{ccr5}_i$, and we define (with $k = 1$ for AIDS and $k = 2$ for SI)

$$\text{ccrAIDS}_i = Z_{1,i} = \begin{cases} Z_i, & \text{if failcode=AIDS} \\ 0, & \text{if failcode=SI} \end{cases}$$

and

$$\text{ccrSI}_i = Z_{2,i} = \begin{cases} 0, & \text{if failcode=AIDS} \\ Z_i, & \text{if failcode=SI} \end{cases}$$

Continuous type-specific variables can be constructed in a similar way. For example, if we want to investigate the effect of age on both cause-specific hazards, we create two columns **ageAIDS** and **ageSI**. The column **ageAIDS** has the value of age if the event type in **failcode** has the value `AIDS` and has value zero otherwise; **ageSI** has the value of age if the event type in **failcode** is `SI` and has value zero otherwise.

Performing the analysis for all event types at once allows for great flexibility in model specification. The major issue is to include the appropriate covariables. Often, a good start is to first create the type-specific variables. In the remaining of this section we give some examples of how covariables are chosen and interpreted for our very simple setting with only two competing risks and one dichotomous covariable. In Sections 4.5 and 4.6 we extend this to much more complicated settings.

If we want to assume that there is no effect of the CCR5 genotype on the progression to SI as the first event, we simply leave out the **ccrSI** covariable.

We can test whether the effects of **ccrAIDS** and **ccrSI** are equal via the null hypothesis that both parameters are equal. An alternative is to use a different contrast and replace one of the type-specific covariables by the original `ccr5` variable. We write

```
coxph(Surv(time,status) ~ ccr5 + ccrSI + strata(failcode),
                                                    aidssi.stack)
```

and obtain

```
           coef exp(coef) se(coef)     z     p
ccr5WM -1.236     0.291     0.307 -4.02 5.7e-05
ccrSI   0.982     2.669     0.389  2.53 1.2e-02
```

This is the same output as when using the CCR5-by-stratum interaction on Page 147. If we use `ccrAIDS` instead of `ccrSI`, we obtain the value $\beta_1 = -0.254$ for the effect on the SI-specific hazard, and the value $\beta_2 = -0.982$ for the additional effect on the AIDS-specific hazard.

When creating the type-specific variables and specifying the contrasts in the model, close attention should be given to the interpretation of the parameters. It is recommended to write down the model and investigate, for each combination of covariable and end point, which parameters contribute to the effect size. In this simplest of all models we have

$$\lambda_k(t) = \lambda_{k,0}(t)\exp(\beta_1 \times \texttt{ccr5} + \beta_2 \times \texttt{ccrSI})\,.$$

Table 4.4 gives the hazard for each end point and each value of CCR5.

TABLE 4.4
Hazard for each combination of variable and event type

AIDS; WW	AIDS; WM	SI; WW	SI; WM
$\lambda_{1,0}(t)$	$\lambda_{1,0}(t)\exp(\beta_1)$	$\lambda_{2,0}(t)$	$\lambda_{2,0}(t)\exp(\beta_1 + \beta_2)$

The AIDS-specific hazard for WM relative to WW is $\exp(\beta_1)$; the effect of WM on the SI-specific hazard is $\exp(\beta_1 + \beta_2)$. These effects are relative to the reference value WW *within* the specific event type. The effect of WM on the SI-specific hazard, relative to its effect on the AIDS-specific hazard is

$$\frac{\lambda_2(t\,|\,WM)}{\lambda_1(t\,|\,WM)} = \frac{\lambda_{2,0}(t)}{\lambda_{1,0}(t)}\exp(\beta_2)\,.$$

4.3.3   Effects equal over causes

Using the stacked data format also allows us to *assume* effects to be equal over event types. Although not justified by the results, let's assume that the CCR5-$\Delta 32$ deletion has the same effect on both cause-specific hazards. Since there is only one effect of CCR5, the original variable can be used:

```
coxph(Surv(time, status) ~ ccr5 + strata(failcode),
                                data = aidssi.stack)
```

By using strata, we allow the baseline hazards to be different. The result is

```
          coef exp(coef) se(coef)      z       p
ccr5WM -0.701      0.496    0.186  -3.77 0.00016


Likelihood ratio test=16.5  on 1 df, p=4.97e-05  n= 648,
                                       number of events= 220
   (10 observations deleted due to missingness)
```

The same result is obtained if we use the original `aidssi` data set, without strata, and combine both end points:

```
coxph(Surv(time, status!=0) ~ ccr5, data = aidssi)
```

which gives

```
          coef exp(coef) se(coef)      z       p
ccr5WM -0.701      0.496    0.186  -3.77 0.00016


Likelihood ratio test=16.5  on 1 df, p=4.95e-05  n= 324,
                                       number of events= 220
   (5 observations deleted due to missingness)
```

Both specifications give the same result because the baseline hazards do not play a role in the partial likelihood. In Section 4.4.2 we show this more formally. For prediction we need the estimates of the baseline hazard and we have to use the stacked data. Note that both approaches coincide with respect to standard error only if we use the non-robust form in the combined analysis.

4.3.4 Proportional baseline hazards

We can also assume cause-specific baseline hazards to be proportional. In our example, if `AIDS` is chosen as the reference value, this would entail

$$\lambda_{SI,0}(t) = \lambda_{AIDS,0}(t) \times \exp(\alpha).$$

If the assumption holds, this model has the added value that we obtain a parametric quantification of the relative progression rates to both end points. With $k = 1$ for `AIDS` and $k = 2$ for `SI`, the model can be formulated as

$$\lambda_k(t \mid \mathbf{Z}_i) = \lambda_{1,0}(t) \exp\{\alpha \times (k-1) + \beta_1 \times \texttt{ccrAIDS}_i + \beta_2 \times \texttt{ccrSI}_i\}. \quad (4.2)$$

Although (k-1) in (4.2) is not a covariable but a failcode specification, a model with proportional baseline hazards can be fitted by letting "type of end point" play the role of a covariable. In R we can fit such a model via

```
coxph(Surv(time, status) ~ ccrAIDS + ccrSI + failcode,
                               data = aidssi.stack)
```

The reason why this works is explained in Section 4.4.3. We obtain as output

	coef	exp(coef)	se(coef)	z	p
ccrAIDS	-1.166	0.311	0.306	-3.81	0.00014
ccrSI	-0.332	0.718	0.237	-1.40	0.16000
failcodeSI	-0.184	0.832	0.148	-1.25	0.21000

Likelihood ratio test=21.5 on 3 df, p=8.12e-05 n= 648,
number of events= 220
(10 observations deleted due to missingness)

Again a robust standard error is not needed because every individual has at most one row with an event. Note that there is no longer an equivalent model based on the original `aidssi` data set.

Since we use a standard Cox proportional hazards approach, we can use established methods to test for non-proportionality of the baseline hazards. In R we use the test based on Schoenfeld residuals as implemented via the `cox.zph` function, which yields:

	rho	chisq	p
ccrAIDS	0.0638	0.885	0.3469
ccrSI	0.0345	0.258	0.6114
failcodeSI	-0.1661	6.069	0.0138
GLOBAL	NA	8.611	0.0349

The p-value of 0.0138 suggests that proportionality does not hold.

The general model can be formulated as

$$\lambda_k(t \mid \mathbf{Z}_i) = \lambda_0(t) \, \exp\{\alpha_k + \beta_k^\top \mathbf{Z}_i\}\,. \tag{4.3}$$

The reference end point k_0 has $\alpha_{k_0} = 0$. It translates to a model for the overall probability to experience an event type of the form [79]

$$\frac{\mathrm{P}(E = k \mid \mathbf{Z})}{\mathrm{P}(E = k_0 \mid \mathbf{Z})} = \exp\left\{\alpha_k + \beta_k^\top \mathbf{Z} - \beta_{k_0}^\top \mathbf{Z}\right\}\,. \tag{4.4}$$

4.4 Why does the stacked approach work?

4.4.1 Cause as stratum variable

The form of the stratified Cox partial likelihood was explained on Page 40. If the effects of all covariables are allowed to differ by stratum, the partial likelihood of the combined model using the stacked data set is the product of the partial likelihoods of the separate analyses. As an example, we show this for the effect of the CCR5 genotype on progression to AIDS and SI switch as competing first events. Let $\boldsymbol{\beta} = (\beta_1, \beta_2) = (\beta_{\mathrm{AIDS}}, \beta_{\mathrm{SI}})$. We use the model specification via the type-specific variables ccrAIDS and ccrSI. Since we used the type of end point as a stratum variable, we have

$$L(\boldsymbol{\beta}) = L^{\text{AIDS}}(\boldsymbol{\beta}) \times L^{\text{SI}}(\boldsymbol{\beta}).$$

The first term $L^{\text{AIDS}}(\boldsymbol{\beta})$ in (4.5) is a product of terms as in (1.29) over the odd rows in aidssi.stack for which **failcode** is equal to AIDS. In these rows, **ccrSI** is always zero. $R_{\text{AIDS}}(t)$ is the set of individuals that are still at risk at time t. It is the same as the risk set $R(t)$ of individuals in aidssi that are still at risk at time t, because the event times have been duplicated in the stacked data set. Furthermore, **ccrAIDS** and **ccr5** have the same value in these rows[3]. Therefore, the expression can be rewritten as the partial likelihood based on the original data set aidssi, with AIDS as the end point, as given in (4.6). Note that in (4.6) we could equivalently write **cause**$_i$ = AIDS instead of **status**$_i = 1$.

$$L^{\text{AIDS}}(\boldsymbol{\beta}) = \prod_{\substack{i=1,3,5,\dots \\ \text{status}_i=1}}^{647} \left\{ \frac{\exp(\beta_1 \times \text{ccrAIDS}_i + \beta_2 \times 0)}{\sum_{j \in R_{\text{AIDS}}(t_i)} \exp(\beta_1 \times \text{ccrAIDS}_j + \beta_2 \times 0)} \right\} \quad (4.5)$$

$$= \prod_{\substack{i=1 \\ \text{status}_i=1}}^{324} \left\{ \frac{\exp(\beta_1 \times \text{ccr5}_i)}{\sum_{j \in R(t_i)} \exp(\beta_1 \times \text{ccr5}_j)} \right\}. \quad (4.6)$$

A similar equality holds for the SI stratum:

$$L^{\text{SI}}(\boldsymbol{\beta}) = \prod_{\substack{i=2,4,6,\dots \\ \text{status}_i=1}}^{648} \left\{ \frac{\exp(\beta_1 \times 0 + \beta_2 \times \text{ccrSI}_i)}{\sum_{j \in R_{\text{SI}}(t_i)} \exp(\beta_1 \times 0 + \beta_2 \times \text{ccrSI}_j)} \right\}$$

$$= \prod_{\substack{i=1 \\ \text{status}_i=2}}^{324} \left\{ \frac{\exp(\beta_2 \times \text{ccr5}_i)}{\sum_{j \in R(t_i)} \exp(\beta_2 \times \text{ccr5}_j)} \right\}.$$

Note that SI as the event is denoted by a value 2 for the **status** variable in the aidssi data set.

The partial likelihood of the combined model is the product of two terms that have no parameters in common, and each of them is the same as the partial likelihood of the corresponding separate model. Therefore, maximisation gives the same paramater values.

The same holds for the null models, i.e. the models in which the parameters are set to the value zero. The likelihood ratio test statistic is twice the difference between the log-likelihood evaluated at the maximum-likelihood estimate and the log-likelihood of the null model. Hence the value of the likelihood ratio test statistic of the combined model is the sum of the likelihood ratio test statistics of the two separate models.

---

[3] Apart from the coding as categorical variable with levels WW and WM or as dummy 0-1 variable.

4.4.2 Effects equal over causes

If we assume that the effect of every covariable is the same for all end points, the analysis based on the stacked data has an equivalent analysis that uses the original data. We show this for the CCR5 example by comparing the partial likelihoods. As in (4.5) and (4.6), the first term in the stratified partial likelihood with the stacked data (4.7) can be rewritten as (4.8), which uses the original data set:

$$L^{\text{AIDS}}(\boldsymbol{\beta}) = \prod_{\substack{i=1,3,5,\dots \\ \text{status}_i=1}}^{647} \left(\frac{\exp(\beta \times \text{ccr5}_i)}{\sum_{j \in R_{\text{AIDS}}(t_i)} \exp(\beta \times \text{ccr5}_j)} \right) \qquad (4.7)$$

$$= \prod_{\substack{i=1 \\ \text{status}_i=1}}^{324} \left(\frac{\exp(\beta \times \text{ccr5}_i)}{\sum_{j \in R(t_i)} \exp(\beta \times \text{ccr5}_j)} \right). \qquad (4.8)$$

A similar relation holds for the second term

$$L^{\text{SI}}(\boldsymbol{\beta}) = \prod_{\substack{i=2,4,6,\dots \\ \text{status}_i=1}}^{648} \left(\frac{\exp(\beta \times \text{ccr5}_i)}{\sum_{j \in R_{\text{SI}}(t_i)} \exp(\beta \times \text{ccr5}_j)} \right)$$

$$= \prod_{\substack{i=1 \\ \text{status}_i=2}}^{324} \left(\frac{\exp(\beta \times \text{ccr5}_i)}{\sum_{j \in R(t_i)} \exp(\beta \times \text{ccr5}_j)} \right). \qquad (4.9)$$

Combining (4.8) and (4.9) yields the partial likelihood based on the original data

$$\prod_{\substack{i=1 \\ \text{status}_i>0}}^{324} \left(\frac{\exp(\beta \times \text{ccr5}_i)}{\sum_{j \in R(t_i)} \exp(\beta \times \text{ccr5}_j)} \right),$$

Because partial likelihoods are the same, all estimates and test statistics are the same as well.

4.4.3 Proportional baseline hazards

A partial likelihood is as a product, over the observed event times, of conditional probabilities that the observed event type happened, given that there was an event observed. As an example, we use the model with type-specific covariables **ccrAIDS** and **ccrSI**. The probability for individual j to have an event of type AIDS at time $t_{(i)}$, given that he was at risk, is $\lambda_{1,0}(t_{(i)}) \exp(\beta_1 \times \text{ccrAIDS}_j)$; for an event of type SI it is $\lambda_{1,0}(t_{(i)}) \exp(\alpha) \exp(\beta_2 \times \text{ccrSI}_j)$. This is the numerator. The denominator is the probability that there is an event among the individuals in the risk set. It consists of two terms, the probability that AIDS occurs and the probability that SI occurs. The contribution to the partial likelihood for the observation at $t_{(i)}$ is

$$\frac{\lambda_{1,0}(t_{(i)})\{\exp(\beta_1 \times \texttt{ccrAIDS}_j)\}^{I(k=1)}\{\exp(\alpha) \times \exp(\beta_2 \times \texttt{ccrSI}_j)\}^{I(k=2)}}{\lambda_{1,0}(t_{(i)}) \sum_{l \in R(t_{(i)})} [\exp\{\beta_1 \times \texttt{ccrAIDS}_l\} + \exp(\alpha) \times \exp\{\beta_2 \times \texttt{ccrSI}_l\}]}$$

The baseline hazards cancel, and we end up with the expression that is maximized in model (4.2).

If we assume the effect of the CCR5-Δ32 deletion to be equal for both event types, then the terms in the partial likelihood can be split into:

$$\frac{\exp(\alpha)^{I(k=2)}}{1 + \exp(\alpha)} \times \frac{\exp(\beta \times \texttt{ccr5}_j)}{\sum_{l \in R(t_{(i)})} \exp(\beta \times \texttt{ccr5}_l)}$$

The second term is the conditional probability that the observed event, of whatever type, was from individual i. The first term is the probability that the event was of the observed type based on the logistic regression specification

$$\text{logit}\{\text{P}(E = SI|\texttt{ccr5}_i)\} = \alpha. \tag{4.10}$$

This is a special case of relation (4.4), which we show to hold for our example. Using relation (2.4) we can write, with $\Lambda_k(t) = \int_0^t \lambda_k(s)ds$ and $\mathbf{Z} = \texttt{ccr5}$,

$$\text{P}(E = \texttt{AIDS} \,|\, \mathbf{Z}) = \int_0^\infty \lambda_{\text{AIDS}}(s|\mathbf{Z}) \exp\big[-\{\Lambda_{\text{AIDS}}(s|\mathbf{Z}) + \Lambda_{\text{SI}}(s|\mathbf{Z})\}\big]ds$$

$$\text{P}(E = \texttt{SI} \,|\, \mathbf{Z}) = \int_0^\infty \lambda_{\text{SI}}(s|\mathbf{Z}) \exp[-\{\Lambda_{\text{AIDS}}(s|\mathbf{Z}) + \Lambda_{\text{SI}}(s|\mathbf{Z})\}]ds.$$

Only the first term in the integrand differs. The proportionality gives

$$\begin{aligned}\lambda_{\text{SI}}(s|\mathbf{Z}) &= \lambda_{1,0}(s)\exp\{\alpha\}\exp\{\beta_2\mathbf{Z}\} \\ &= \exp\{\alpha\}\exp\{(\beta_2 - \beta_1)\mathbf{Z}\} \times \lambda_{1,0}(s)\exp\{\beta_1\mathbf{Z}\} \\ &= \exp\{\alpha\}\exp\{(\beta_2 - \beta_1)\mathbf{Z}\} \times \lambda_{\text{AIDS}}(s|\mathbf{Z}),\end{aligned}$$

and we obtain

$$\text{P}(E = \texttt{SI} \,|\, \mathbf{Z}) = \exp\{\alpha + (\beta_2 - \beta_1)\mathbf{Z}\} \times \text{P}(E = \texttt{AIDS} \,|\, \mathbf{Z}).$$

4.5 Multi-state regression models for transition hazards

When quantifying the effect of covariables on the transition hazard in a multi-state setting, the same modeling choices can be made as in a competing risks setting. We can specify and fit a proportional transition hazards model separately for every transition. However, often it is more interesting or even necessary to make further assumptions. For such analyses we need a stacked data set. The stacked data format combines the data that are used for the analysis per transition. It has one row per transition for which an individual has been at risk, including transitions that were not observed because a competing one occurred. This is different from the transition-based data format that was described in Section 3.4.1, which has one row per *observed* transition.

As an example we use the multi-state model that was described in Figure 3.3. It additionally considers what happens after AIDS or SI as the first event. For example, we can investigate whether the effect of the CCR5-Δ32 deletion on progression changes after the virus has switched to the SI phenotype. If the SI phenotype can use another receptor for cell entry, having the deletion may no longer be advantageous.

We use the `aidssi2` data set that was described in Section 3.4.1. In Table 4.5 we show the four individuals from Table 3.1 in the stacked format. The columns **Tstart** and **Tstop** give the time of entry into and exit from the state in **from**. There is a row for every possible state **to** that can be reached from **from**. The column with the transition number, **trans**, plays the same role as the **failcode** column in Table 4.2. We use the state values as required by the `mstate` package; they are all shifted by one compared to Figure 3.3.

TABLE 4.5
Time and status information in stacked long format for four individuals from `aidssi2` data set

row	patnr	from	to	trans	Tstart	Tstop	time	status
49	14	1	2	1	0	5.05	5.05	0
50	14	1	3	2	0	5.05	5.05	0
7	3	1	2	1	1.81	2.23	0.43	1
8	3	1	3	2	1.81	2.23	0.43	0
9	3	2	4	3	2.23	2.26	0.02	0
10	3	2	5	4	2.23	2.26	0.02	1
51	15	1	2	1	1.80	10.20	8.39	1
52	15	1	3	2	1.80	10.20	8.39	0
53	15	2	4	3	10.20	12.93	2.74	0
54	15	2	5	4	10.20	12.93	2.74	0
26	8	1	2	1	2.80	8.61	5.80	0
27	8	1	3	2	2.80	8.61	5.80	1
28	8	3	4	5	8.61	11.46	2.85	1
29	8	4	5	6	11.46	11.94	0.48	1

Since individual 14 did not experience any of the events, he only has two rows: one for AIDS and one for SI as the possible next state. Individual 3 entered the study at 1.81 years after HIV infection. He developed AIDS at 2.23 years, as can be seen by the **status** value of 1 in the row with **trans** equal to 1. From that moment onwards, he became at risk for the transitions that can occur from state 2, namely transition number 3 to state AIDS/SI and transition 4 to the absorbing death state. Transition 4 was observed at 2.26 years after HIV infection. Transient states 3 and 4 were never reached and hence do not occur in **from**. Individual 15 developed AIDS at 10.20 years, after which he was at risk for the same transitions 3 and 4 as individual 3, but he remained in state 2 until his last observation. Hence, he has the **status** variable equal to 0 in both rows that refer to the transitions from state 2. Individual 8 progressed to death via the upper path in Figure 3.3. Since only one transition is possible from states 3 and 4, he contributes 4 rows to the data set. Note that, contrary to the competing risks setting, individuals may have several rows with the status variable equal to 1.

Each transition can be analyzed separately by selecting the rows that have the **trans** variable equal to that transition. The output from the six separate proportional transition hazards models is shown in Table 4.6. The effect of the CCR5-Δ32 deletion on the transition rates from the initial state to SI and AIDS are comparable to the estimates on Page 148[4]. We also included age at HIV infection, which is in the **age.inf** column.

TABLE 4.6
Effects of CCR5-Δ32 deletion and age at infection (per 10 years)

	trans	var	coef	RH	se(coef)	z	p.value
1.	HIV → AIDS	ccr5WM	−1.14	0.32	0.30	−3.83	<0.001
		age.inf	0.22	1.24	0.14	1.56	0.12
2.	HIV → SI	ccr5WM	−0.21	0.81	0.24	−0.87	0.38
		age.inf	0.12	1.12	0.14	0.83	0.41
3.	AIDS → AIDS/SI	ccr5WM	−18.06	0.00	13151.59	−0.00	1.00
		age.inf	−0.21	0.81	0.66	−0.32	0.75
4.	AIDS → death	ccr5WM	−0.10	0.91	0.38	−0.26	0.79
		age.inf	0.19	1.21	0.15	1.25	0.21
5.	SI → AIDS/SI	ccr5WM	−0.48	0.62	0.29	−1.66	0.10
		age.inf	0.17	1.18	0.15	1.13	0.26
6.	AIDS/SI → death	ccr5WM	0.36	1.43	0.32	1.14	0.25
		age.inf	0.24	1.27	0.18	1.30	0.19

When looking at the output, we make the following observations:

1. Only the effect of the CCR5-Δ32 deletion on progression from HIV infection to AIDS is significant.

2. Individuals with the CCR5-Δ32 deletion have a smaller transition hazard for both transitions on the pathway HIV → SI → AIDS.

3. The estimated effect of the CCR5-Δ32 deletion on the transition from AIDS to AIDS/SI is very strong, but at the same time with a huge standard error, resulting in a non-significant p-value.

4. The effect of age at infection is never significant, but most relative hazards have about the same size. Except for transition 4, all relative hazards are between 1.12 and 1.27 per 10 year increase in age at infection.

---

[4]They are not exactly the same due to some small changes we made in the data set and the inclusion of age as a covariable.

The reason for observation 3 is that only 6 men had a switch to SI after AIDS diagnosis (see Table 3.3). All these men had the wild type WW of the CCR5 encoding gene. Therefore, there was no contrast for this transition and the Wald test cannot be used (we could use the likelihood ratio test). If we want to include both covariables as effects on the transition hazard from AIDS to AIDS/SI, an alternative is to assume the effect of the CCR5-Δ32 delection to be equal to its effect on some other transition. The most logical assumption is to make it equal to the effect on the other transition to SI, HIV → SI. Because of observation 4, we may assume the effect of age to be equal for all transitions. The effect of age was smaller for transition 4, but this was based on only six events and the 95% confidence intervals overlap.

We can only make these assumptions if we use a stacked data format. We create the type-specific covariables; in a multi-state setting we call them transition-specific covariables. We first test whether the effect of age can be assumed the same for all transitions: we compare a model with all transition-specific covariables included with a model that assumes all age effects to be equal. Since the likelihood ratio test has a p-value of 0.96, assuming one overall age effect seems justified.

4.5.1 Combined analyses: assume effects to be equal

With our modeling assumptions we use a set of covariables as in Table 4.7. For **ccr5** we create five transition-specific covariables. One, **ccr5.23**, is for the transitions 2 and 3 together. The other four columns are for the transitions 1, 4, 5 and 6. The individuals with the WW genotype have the value zero in all columns. Individual number 15, who has WM, has the variable **ccr5.23** equal

TABLE 4.7

Information on age and transition-specific CCR5 covariables from four example individuals in the `aidssi2` data set

patnr	trans	age.inf	ccr5	ccr5.23	ccr5.1	ccr5.4	ccr5.5	ccr5.6
14	1	34.9	WW	0	0	0	0	0
14	2	34.9	WW	0	0	0	0	0
3	1	39.0	WW	0	0	0	0	0
3	2	39.0	WW	0	0	0	0	0
3	3	39.0	WW	0	0	0	0	0
3	4	39.0	WW	0	0	0	0	0
15	1	26.8	WM	0	1	0	0	0
15	2	26.8	WM	1	0	0	0	0
15	3	26.8	WM	1	0	0	0	0
15	4	26.8	WM	0	0	1	0	0
8	1	30.8	WW	0	0	0	0	0
8	2	30.8	WW	0	0	0	0	0
8	5	30.8	WW	0	0	0	0	0
8	6	30.8	WW	0	0	0	0	0

to 1 in both his second and third row, which refer to the transitions 2 and 3. Similarly, **ccr5.1** and **ccr5.4** have the value 1 in the rows that refer to these transitions. For age we can use the original variable.

We use **trans** as a stratum variable to allow for separate baseline hazards per transition. Writing

```
fit.aidssi.mst <- coxph(Surv(Tstart,Tstop,status) ~
    strata(trans) + ccr5.23 + ccr5.1 + ccr5.4 + ccr5.5 + ccr5.6
                            + I(age.inf/10), data=aidssi.mst)
```

we obtain as parameter estimates

	coef	exp(coef)	se(coef)	z	p
ccr5.23	-0.2237	0.800	0.2378	-0.941	0.34689
ccr5.1	-1.1454	0.318	0.2963	-3.866	0.00011
ccr5.4	-0.0943	0.910	0.3725	-0.253	0.80007
ccr5.5	-0.4830	0.617	0.2883	-1.675	0.09386
ccr5.6	0.3731	1.452	0.3131	1.192	0.23341
I(age.inf/10)	0.1748	1.191	0.0669	2.613	0.00899

We can see the power of the stacked approach in the effect of age at infection. By combining information over all transitions, it has become significant, even though the parameter estimate itself hardly changed compared to the separate analyses. Of course, this gain in power is under the condition that all age effects are approximately the same. The effects of the CCR5-Δ32 deletion are comparable with the ones for transitions 1, 2, 4, 5 and 6 from the separate model fits in Table 4.6. Although not significant, both effects of WM on the pathway HIV $\rightarrow$ SI $\rightarrow$ AIDS are below one. We investigate whether the deletion affects this pathway by testing the null hypothesis H_0:ccr5.23=ccr5.5=0. We use a model in which we leave out the covariables ccr5.23 and ccr5.5 and compare the fits via the likelihood ratio test. The p-value of 0.13 gives no convincing evidence of an effect via this pathway.

4.5.2 Proportional baseline hazards

In the previous analyses we assumed every transition to have its own baseline hazard which we left completely unspecified. Based on the fitted model, we compute the Breslow estimate of the cumulative baseline hazards. In Figure 4.2 it is shown for all six transitions. They are the cumulative hazards when the covariables are set at their mean value. The shape of the curve does not depend on the covariable combination (see Page 39). The large jumps in the beginning don't cause problems for the parameter estimates, because events that occur when few individuals are at risk receive less weight.

The curves resemble the ones from the nonparametric analysis (Figure 3.4). The increase in the cumulative baseline hazards is much larger for the transitions SI $\rightarrow$ AIDS/SI, AIDS $\rightarrow$ death and AIDS/SI $\rightarrow$ death. We would like to quantify via a parameter how much larger they are. If baseline hazards are

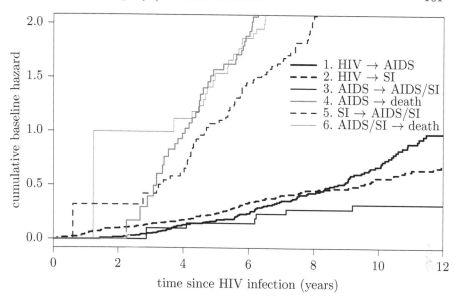

FIGURE 4.2
Estimated baseline hazards for all six transitions.

more or less proportional, we can do this by including transition type as a categorical covariable instead of as a stratum. We fit the model

$$\lambda_k(t \mid \mathbf{Z}_i) = \lambda_{2,0}(t) \, \exp(\alpha_k + \beta_k^\top \texttt{ccr5} + \gamma \times \texttt{age.inf}). \qquad (4.11)$$

We write $\beta_k^\top \texttt{ccr5}$ as a shorthand notation for the transition-specific effects of CCR5. We estimate five parameters α_k for the effect of transition type. Since the first transition HIV → AIDS crosses two of the other curves, its effect may not be proportional to the others. We therefore choose HIV → SI as the reference transition, implying that $\alpha_2 = 0$, and we test for proportionality relative to this transition. We fit the model via[5]

```
fit.aidssi.mst2 <- coxph(Surv(Tstart,Tstop,status) ~
        relevel(trans,2) + ccr5.23 + ccr5.1 + ccr5.4 + ccr5.5
                + ccr5.6 + I(age.inf/10), data=aidssi.mst)
```

We test whether the proportionality assumption is justified by using the Schoenfeld residuals from the model fit:

```
cox.zph(fit.aidssi.csh2)
```

---

[5]In R, the first level of a categorical variable of class *factor* is the default reference value. This is transition 1. We use the `relevel` function to make transition 2 the reference.

This yields the following result[6]:

	rho	chisq	p
trans1	0.1238	7.5637	0.00596
trans3	-0.0526	1.3739	0.24114
trans4	0.0312	0.4717	0.49221
trans5	0.0388	0.7317	0.39234
trans6	0.0687	2.2368	0.13476
ccr5.23	0.0147	0.1065	0.74421
ccr5.1	0.0509	1.2841	0.25714
ccr5.4	-0.0300	0.4746	0.49089
ccr5.5	-0.0322	0.5265	0.46806
ccr5.6	0.0294	0.4184	0.51774
I(age.inf/10)	0.0124	0.0809	0.77615
GLOBAL	NA	18.3024	0.07482

The global test for non-proportionality is not significant at the 0.05 level. However, based on Figure 4.2 and the p-value of 0.006, we do not want to make the proportionality assumption for the transition HIV → AIDS. If we make transition 1 the reference transition, non-proportionality is also suggested for the transitions 3, 4 and 5, with p-values of 0.033, 0.051 and 0.093 respectively. Hence transition 1 is the one that most clearly deviates.

Therefore, we fit a proportional transition hazards model with two baseline hazards, one for transition HIV → AIDS and one for all other transitions. We create two variables, which are shown in Table 4.8, for our example individuals. The variable **tr.AIDS** separates transition 1 from the rest and is used as

TABLE 4.8

Information on time and transition for four example individuals; covariables **tr.AIDS** and **tr.prop** are used to parametrize baseline hazards

patnr	from	to	trans	tr.AIDS	tr.prop	Tstart	Tstop	status
49	14	1 2	1	1	2	0.00	5.05	0
50	14	1 3	2	2	2	0.00	5.05	0
7	3	1 2	1	1	2	1.81	2.23	1
8	3	1 3	2	2	2	1.81	2.23	0
9	3	2 4	3	2	3	2.23	2.26	0
10	3	2 5	4	2	4	2.23	2.26	1
51	15	1 2	1	1	2	1.80	10.20	1
52	15	1 3	2	2	2	1.80	10.20	0
53	15	2 4	3	2	3	10.20	12.93	0
54	15	2 5	4	2	4	10.20	12.93	0
26	8	1 2	1	1	2	2.80	8.61	0
27	8	1 3	2	2	2	2.80	8.61	1
28	8	3 4	5	2	5	8.61	11.46	1
29	8	4 5	6	2	6	11.46	11.94	1

---

[6]The true row labels in the output are `relevel(trans, 2)1` etcetera.

stratum variable. The column **tr.prop** is used for the transitions that we assume to have proportional baseline hazards. Transition 1 needs a value in this column as well. Any value is fine, as long as it is the same value for all. This is because a value that is constant in a stratum does not contribute to the likelihood (the same was observed in Section 4.4.1). We choose to give it the value 2 of the reference transition.

The model is fitted via

```
fit.aidssi.mst3 <- coxph(Surv(Tstart,Tstop,status) ~
    strata(tr.AIDS) + tr.prop + ccr5.23 + ccr5.1 +
    ccr5.4 + ccr5.5 + ccr5.6 + I(age.inf/10), data=aidssi.mst)
```

and we obtain

	coef	exp(coef)	se(coef)	z	p
tr.prop3	-0.7304	0.482	0.424	-1.723	0.08490
tr.prop4	2.0268	7.590	0.162	12.507	0.00000
tr.prop5	1.5724	4.818	0.166	9.491	0.00000
tr.prop6	2.2326	9.324	0.172	12.966	0.00000
ccr5.23	-0.2674	0.765	0.236	-1.135	0.25635
ccr5.1	-1.1429	0.319	0.296	-3.857	0.00011
ccr5.4	-0.0888	0.915	0.357	-0.249	0.80372
ccr5.5	-0.4937	0.610	0.286	-1.725	0.08456
ccr5.6	0.3758	1.456	0.297	1.264	0.20629
I(age.inf/10)	0.1886	1.208	0.066	2.860	0.00424

When interpreting the parameter estimates, it may be of help to use a schematic representation as in Table 4.9. For each of the transitions 1, 2,..., 6, it is shown whether the covariable contributes via an "o". For example, ccr5.23 contributes to transitions 2 and 3 and age.inf contributes to all transitions. In this example the relation between parameter and transition is still rather straightforward, but in more complicated model formulations as in

TABLE 4.9
Schematic description of covariable effects in `fit.aidssi.mst3`

	1	2	3	4	5	6	estimate
tr.prop3: AIDS → AIDS/SI			o				−0.7304
tr.prop4: AIDS → death				o			2.0268
tr.prop5: SI → AIDS/SI					o		1.5724
tr.prop6: AIDS/SI → death						o	2.2326
ccr5.23 SI switch		o	o				−0.2674
ccr5.1: HIV → AIDS	o						−1.1429
ccr5.4: AIDS → death				o			−0.0888
ccr5.5: SI → AIDS/SI					o		−0.4937
ccr5.6: AIDS/SI → death						o	0.3758
age.inf	o	o	o	o	o	o	0.1886

Section 4.6, such a table is very insightful when we want to quantify relative hazards for different combinations of covariables (see Figure 4.7).

Relative baseline hazards are in correspondence with Figure 4.2. Transition 3 has a 0.48 times smaller baseline hazard than transition 2, whereas the other three transitions have significantly larger baseline hazards. The effect of the covariables does not change much compared to the model that uses a separate baseline hazard for every transition. This is what we expect to happen if the proportionality assumption is reasonable.

Assuming proportionality is a useful tool to compare rates for different transitions via simple parameters. Proportional baseline hazards may have little biological justification. Yet, we make the same assumption if we quantify the effect of a dichotomous time-varying covariable in a proportional hazards model. In Section 4.5.3 we explain that this is the same as assuming proportionality of baseline hazards for transitions to the same incoming state.

4.5.3   Dual role of intermediate states

Intermediate states play a dual role in multi-state models. Entrance into the state can be seen as an event that can occur from an earlier state, but also as a change in a covariable that affects the transition rate to a subsequent state [79].

For example, on the pathway from HIV infection to AIDS, an individual may first experience a switch to SI. State SI plays the role of event if we concentrate on transitions 1 and 2 out of the HIV state in Figure 4.3. It plays the role of time-varying covariable if we compare transitions 1 and 5: a switch to SI may impact the AIDS hazard.

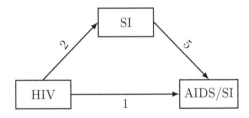

FIGURE 4.3
Illness-death model for the effect of the SI switch on the pathway to AIDS.

The effect of a time-varying covariable in a proportional hazards model is typically quantified via a parameter. In the multi-state setting of our example, this entails that we assume the baseline hazards for transitions 1 and 5 to be proportional. If we have doubts about the proportionality assumption and the covariable is categorical, an alternative is to include it as a stratum variable. Then a separate baseline hazard is modeled for each value of the covariable.

In our example this entails that we allow transitions 1 and 5 to have their own baseline hazard.

It will come as no surprise that the stacked data set already has the correct structure for modeling the effect of time-varying covariables. We explained in Section 1.8.5 that the effect of time-varying covariables on the hazard can be modeled by splitting the follow-up time over different rows when the value of the variable changes. Example individual 8 in Table 4.5 experienced a switch to SI as the first event at 8.61 years after HIV infection. Rows 27 and 28 describe this updated information on SI switch before AIDS. The change in the SI covariable is represented by the values 1 and 3 in column **from** (or equivalently by the values 2 and 5 in column **trans**). The effect of the SI switch to AIDS progression is quantified by comparing such individuals with the ones that did not have an SI switch. In individuals 3 and 15, who developed AIDS without having had an SI switch before, the information on time to AIDS is contained in a single row (rows 7 and 51). In individual 14, who was censored in the HIV state, we can use either of the two rows 49 and 50. If we include transition as a covariable, we assume proportionality and we quantify the effect of the SI switch on the AIDS hazard via a parameter. The effect of the switch to SI is modeled via

```
coxph(Surv(Tstart,Tstop,status) ~ trans, data=aidssi.mst,
                                  subset=trans %in% c(1,5))
```

and we obtain[7]

```
       coef exp(coef) se(coef)    z  p
trans5 1.33      3.77    0.146 9.08  0
```

But we can also allow the effect of the SI switch on progression to AIDS to be non-proportional by using **trans** as a stratum variable.

4.5.4 Beyond the Markov model: effect of transition time

Until now we have performed the analyses under the Markov assumption that the transition hazard only depends on the state that is occupied and the value of the covariables, not on the transition history. One way to relax this assumption is by allowing the transition hazard to depend on the time at which a state is reached.

As an example, we investigate whether progression to death after AIDS depends on how long after HIV infection AIDS develops. We assume the death hazard only to depend on the time of the AIDS diagnosis, not on the pathway along which AIDS was reached. For this, we create a variable **aids.time**. For the rows that have death as the incoming state it has as value the time of the AIDS diagnosis. For the other rows it has the value zero. This value zero is fairly arbitrary; the only thing that matters is that the value is the same over

---

[7]The effects table has four more rows with missing values, which refer to the other transitions.

all rows (see Exercise 2 in Section 4.8). For our example individuals, it has
the values as in Table 4.10. Individual number 3 developed AIDS before an
SI switch at 2.23 years after HIV infection. From state AIDS, he is at risk for
transitions 3 to SI switch and 5 to death. We assume that the time of AIDS
only affects the transition hazard to death, not to SI. Therefore, only the row
that refers to transition 5 has the value 2.23. The same holds for individual
15. Individual 8 developed AIDS after an SI switch at time 11.46 and this
value is assigned to the row that refers to transition 6.

TABLE 4.10
Information on time and transition for four example
individuals; covariable **aids.time** gives time of AIDS

patnr	from	to	trans	Tstart	Tstop	status	aids.time
49	14	1	2	1	0.00	5.05	0	0.00
50	14	1	3	2	0.00	5.05	0	0.00
7	3	1	2	1	1.81	2.23	1	0.00
8	3	1	3	2	1.81	2.23	0	0.00
9	3	2	4	3	2.23	2.26	0	0.00
10	3	2	5	4	2.23	2.26	1	2.23
51	15	1	2	1	1.80	10.20	1	0.00
52	15	1	3	2	1.80	10.20	0	0.00
53	15	2	4	3	10.20	12.93	0	0.00
54	15	2	5	4	10.20	12.93	0	10.20
26	8	1	2	1	2.80	8.61	0	0.00
27	8	1	3	2	2.80	8.61	1	0.00
28	8	3	4	5	8.61	11.46	1	0.00
29	8	4	5	6	11.46	11.94	1	11.46

We add **aids.time** to the model:

```
fit.aidssi.mst4 <- coxph(Surv(Tstart,Tstop,status) ~
    strata(tr.AIDS) + tr.prop + ccr5.23 + ccr5.1 + ccr5.4 +
    ccr5.5 + ccr5.6 + I(age.inf/10) + aids.time, data=aidssi.mst)
```

The effect of the time of AIDS diagnosis on mortality is

```
            coef exp(coef) se(coef)      z        p
aids.time  0.019     1.019   0.0372  0.511 6.1e-01
```

The other effects change very little. We conclude that there is no reason to
assume that this violation of the Markov assumption holds. However, there
may be other ways in which the Markov assumption is violated. The transition
hazard to death may depend on time *since* AIDS diagnosis instead of time *at*
AIDS diagnosis, which would require us to incorporate an extra time scale. Or
a transition hazard may depend on which previous states have been visited.
For example, the transition hazard from AIDS/SI to death may depend on
the pathway from HIV to AIDS/SI. Or there may be individual frailties that
make some individuals progress through the different states more rapidly than

others [82]. This causes individual transition times to subsequent states to be correlated.

4.5.5 Standard error

In the competing risks setting, individuals have at most one transition. Therefore, a robust estimator of the standard error is not needed. In the multi-state setting this is less clear-cut. If we stack the data but fit models with separate baseline hazards and covariable effects per transition, we maximize the same partial likelihood as when one model per transition is fitted. The usual non-robust estimator is the same as in the separate models. If we assume effects to be equal over transitions or if we assume proportional baseline hazards, an individual can contribute more than one event to a parameter estimate. Use of a robust estimator has been suggested [100, Section 8.6]. If the Markov assumption holds, what happens next only depends on the covariables and the current state and transitions from the same individual are unrelated. Still, it may be a safe option to use a sandwich estimator, although it tends to be more variable. At the other extreme is the situation with repeated events of the same type, in which the presence of a correlation between events from the same individual is likely.

If we use a robust standard error in the model from Section 4.5.1, the standard error and p-value change slightly:

	coef	se(coef)		robust se	robust p
ccr5.23	-0.2237	0.2378	0.34689	0.2319	0.33485
ccr5.1	-1.1454	0.2963	0.00011	0.2815	0.00005
ccr5.4	-0.0943	0.3725	0.80007	0.4055	0.81600
ccr5.5	-0.4830	0.2883	0.09386	0.2310	0.03651
ccr5.6	0.3731	0.3131	0.23341	0.2529	0.14020
I(age.inf/10)	0.1748	0.0669	0.00899	0.0665	0.00854

The robust estimator is equal to the working independence estimator in generalized estimating equations (GEE) models [67]. An alternative is to use a frailty term. Note that GEE and frailty models have different interpretations of the parameters. A GEE model is a marginal model, whereas a frailty model is a conditional model [49]).

4.6 Example: causes of death in HIV infected individuals

We investigate the effect of the introduction of cART and of HCV infection on the spectrum in causes of death in HIV infected individuals (see Example 2 in Section 1.2.2). HCV can cause liver problems, which may ultimately lead to death. Its effect on other causes of death (COD) is uncertain. We perform a competing risks analysis, discriminating among four CODs: i) liver related mortality, ii) AIDS related mortality, iii) natural causes (e.g. due to cardio-vascular disease and cancer) and iv) non-natural causes (accident, overdose, suicide) [104]. We use data on 9164 individuals from 16 cohort studies participating in the CASCADE collaboration [19]. The data covers the period from 1980 until 2007.

HIV infection is chosen as the origin of the principal time scale. HCV infection is included as a time-fixed covariable; all infections are assumed to have occurred before HIV infection. For the effect of cART, we dichotomize the calendar year into the pre-cART period (before 1997) and cART period (1997 and later). We use the calendar period of follow-up, not the calendar period of HIV infection. Hence it is included as a time-varying covariable as was explained on Page 41 and in Figure 1.17 (but now with only two periods). Individuals contribute to both periods if they became HIV infected and entered the study before 1997 and were still alive and in follow-up after 1997. There is right censoring due to loss to follow-up as well as administrative censoring. Furthermore, there are three mechanisms that induce left truncation. First, there was late entry because some individuals entered the study after HIV infection. Second, some cohorts only started to systematically test for HCV status in later calendar years. In order to prevent bias due to selective testing, we only include information from the date that systematic testing was introduced; individuals that died before that date are excluded[8]. Third, since the calendar period of follow-up is a time-varying covariable, individuals can enter the second period after HIV infection (this is internal left truncation; see Section 1.8.5).

The nonparametric estimates of the cause-specific mortality are shown in Figure 4.4, using a separate display format. Note that the range of the y-axis differs per COD. Before 1997, HCV coinfected individuals had higher liver-related mortality and mortality due to non-natural causes, but they had lower AIDS related mortality and mortality due to natural causes. From 1997 onwards, HCV coinfected individuals had higher mortality for three of the four CODs.

Some of the differences by HCV status may be explained by the presence of confounders. For example, the higher non-natural mortality in HCV coinfected individuals may be caused by the large contribution of injecting drug users to the HCV coinfected group. Therefore, we perform a multivariable analysis in which we correct for risk group, gender, and age at HIV infection. These variables are chosen a priori based on background knowledge. Risk group is based on the most likely source of HIV infection and we discriminate between MSM (men who became HIV infected through sex with another man), MSW (HIV infection through sexual contact with the other gender), IDU (HIV infection through injection drug use) and persons with haemophilia who became

---

[8]In analogy to administrative right censoring, we could call this administrative truncation.

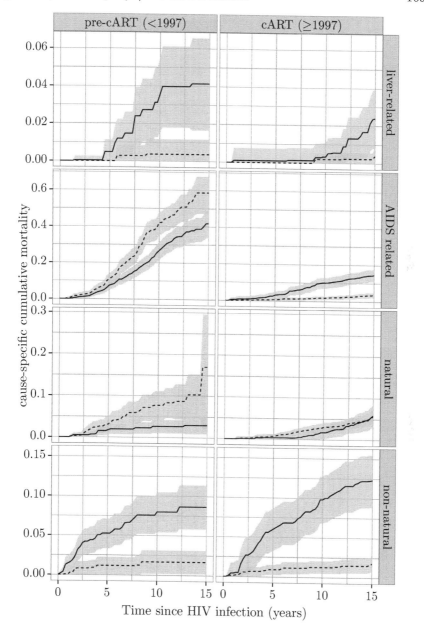

FIGURE 4.4
Cause-specific cumulative mortality by HCV status and calendar period of
follow-up. Dashed line: HIV mono-infected individuals; solid line: HCV/HIV
coinfected individuals. 95% confidence intervals in grey.

infected through blood transfusion. The same three variables may modify the effect of HCV infection and cART period on mortality. For example, IDUs are less likely to receive cART and be adherent, leading to increased AIDS related mortality in the cART period relative to other HIV infected risk groups.

In Figure 4.5 we show the amount of information on overall mortality by risk group and gender for the four combinations of HCV status and calendar period. Some risk groups have a very skewed distribution over the four combinations. For example, the MSW group only contributes 45 person-years of follow-up and one death to the HCV infected group before 1997. Or even more extreme: there are no HCV negative persons with haemophilia. This imposes a problem in our regression model, unless we leave out some of the interaction terms. For example, by leaving out the interaction term between HCV status and risk group, we have $9 + 1 = 10$ deaths and $428 + 45 = 473$ person-years of follow-up in the MSW group in the pre-cART period. Patterns in Figure 4.5 reflect the model on overall mortality that was fitted to these data [104]. Using a Cox model, the effect of HCV coinfection was assumed to be the same for

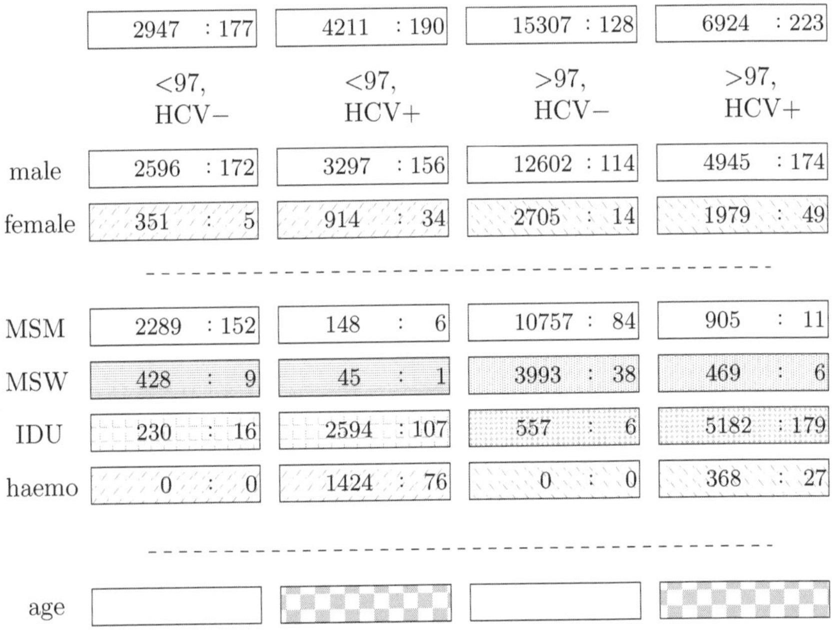

	<97, HCV−	<97, HCV+	>97, HCV−	>97, HCV+
	2947 : 177	4211 : 190	15307 : 128	6924 : 223
male	2596 : 172	3297 : 156	12602 : 114	4945 : 174
female	351 : 5	914 : 34	2705 : 14	1979 : 49
MSM	2289 : 152	148 : 6	10757 : 84	905 : 11
MSW	428 : 9	45 : 1	3993 : 38	469 : 6
IDU	230 : 16	2594 : 107	557 : 6	5182 : 179
haemo	0 : 0	1424 : 76	0 : 0	368 : 27
age				

FIGURE 4.5
Person-years of follow-up (before colon) and number of deaths (after colon) for each combination of HCV status and calendar period, overall and by values of risk group and gender. Rectangles with the same pattern denote combinations for which covariable effects were assumed equal in the regression model for overall survival [104].

both genders and each risk group, while the effect of HCV status was assumed to be the same in both calendar periods.

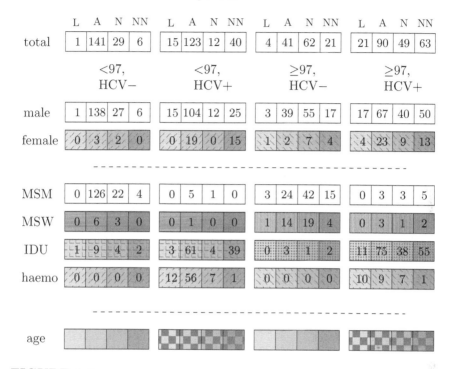

FIGURE 4.6
Number of cause-specific deaths within subgroups by combination of HCV and calendar period. Patterns in rectangles have same meaning as in Figure 4.5. L: liver related; A: AIDS related; N: natural; NN: non-natural.

Here we concentrate on the competing risks analyses. If we split overall mortality into the four CODs, the problem of lack of information is aggravated. Figure 4.6 has the information from Figure 4.5 split up by COD[9]. AIDS was the most frequent COD for three of the four combinations of HCV status and calendar period. Liver related mortality was rare, with only 5 cases in HIV mono-infected individuals. The numbers in Figure 4.6 tell us that we cannot repeat the analysis that we did for overall survival. By splitting up mortality into four different causes, the number of cause-specific deaths for specific covariable values becomes very low or even zero. For example, we have ten deaths to quantify overall mortality in the MSW group in the period before 1997. However, only three of them died of natural causes and none died of non-natural or liver related causes.

---

[9]We left out the person-years of follow-up, because these numbers do not change compared to Figure 4.5.

We can solve this problem by performing the analysis for all CODs in one single model in which we assume the effects of some covariables to be equal for different CODs. For this, we carefully define the contrasts and create the appropriate variables. In the next section, we describe and motivate the modeling choices and summarize the results.

4.6.1   Analysis using well-defined contrasts

The definition of the contrasts determines the interpretation of the parameters. On Page 151 we saw an example: if we use **ccr AIDS**, **ccrSI** quantifies the effect of the deletion on progression to SI; if we use **ccr5**, **ccrSI** quantifies the *additional* effect of the deletion on progression to SI compared to progression to AIDS. The effect of the latter contrast was explained in Table 4.9. In Figure 4.7 we give a similar schematic overview of the contrasts we use in the current model. Every column corresponds to one combination of HCV status, calendar period and COD; there are $2 \times 2 \times 4 = 16$ columns in total. In the final column we give the estimates of the parameter values (on the scale of the log of the relative hazard) and their amount of significance. We choose HIV mono-infected individuals and follow-up period <1997 as the reference group. The first 11 rows quantify the effect of the other combinations of HCV status and calendar period at the reference values of the other covariables, `male` for gender, `MSM` for risk group and 30 years for age at HIV infection[10]. To see whether another value of each of them changes the hazard for a specific HCV/period combination, we look at rows 12 to 26. Hazards for any two combinations of covariables can be compared by looking at the squares that contain an "o". If we want to quantify combination B relative to combination A, we sum the estimates from the rows with an "o" that satisfy B and subtract the sum of the estimates from the rows with an "o" that satisfy A. We give a couple of examples in the next paragraphs; you can try some other combinations in Exercise 4 of Section 4.8.

Baseline hazards

We are primarily interested in the relative progression rates per COD. Therefore, we do not assume proportionality of the cause-specific baseline hazards and we include COD as a stratum variable in the model. As a consequence, there are no parameters in the upper left part of Figure 4.7 (we could also draw a matrix of empty squares).

Effects of HCV coinfection and cART period in reference group

The parameters in rows 1 to 4 in Figure 4.7 quantify the effect of HCV coinfection on each COD in the pre-cART period for the reference group. HCV infection increased the cause-specific hazard for liver related death by

---

[10]Note that MSM are always male.

#		<97, HCV−				<97, HCV+				≥97, HCV−				≥97, HCV+				β
		L	A	N	NN	L	A	N	NN	L	A	N	NN	L	A	N	NN	
1.	HCV					o								o				3.48 **
2.	baseline						o								o			−0.45
3.	hazards							o								o		−1.23 **
4.									o								o	−0.13
5.	≥ 97										o				o			−3.26 ***
6.												o				o		−1.48 ***
7.													o				o	−0.35
8.	HCV													o				−1.17 **
9.	×														o			1.48 ***
10.	≥ 97															o		1.65 ***
11.																	o	0.84
12.	female	o	o	o	o	o	o	o	o	o	o	o	o	o	o	o	o	−0.44 *
13.	× ≥ 97											o	o			o	o	0.01
14.	× ≥ 97									o				o				0.01
15.	msw/haem						o	o	o						o	o	o	0.16
16.	IDU	o				o				o				o				0.18
17.	IDU		o				o				o				o			0.55
18.	IDU			o					o			o					o	2.34 ***
19.	× ≥ 97									o				o				0.48
20.	× ≥ 97											o	o			o	o	−0.52
21.	× HCV					o	o	o						o	o	o		0.26
22.	× HCV								o								o	−0.00
23.	age/10yrs	o	o	o		o	o	o		o	o	o		o	o	o		0.41 ***
24.	age				o				o				o				o	0.25 .
25.	× HCV					o	o	o						o	o	o		0.09
26.	× HCV					o								o				0.36 *

FIGURE 4.7
Covariable combinations chosen in the regression model for the four CODs.
L: liver related; A: AIDS related; N: natural; NN: non-natural.
P-values: $0 < {}^{***} < 0.001 < {}^{**} < 0.01 < {}^{*} < 0.05 < . < 0.1 < \quad < 1$

a factor $\exp(3.48) = 32.5$ and decreased the hazard for natural death by $\exp(-1.23) = 0.29$. For AIDS related death, the hazard decreased by a non-significant factor $\exp(-0.45) = 0.64$. Note that these values should not be interpreted as marginal hazards; if liver related death occurs more often, it may make non-natural death less likely. Also note that there were no liver related deaths observed in MSM. However, we assume the increase to be the same as in MSW and in persons with haemophilia[11].

The parameters in rows 5 to 7 quantify the change in hazard after the introduction of cART for HIV mono-infected individuals. Since there were only 5 HIV mono-infected individuals that died of liver related causes, we assume liver related mortality in this group to be the same in both calendar periods: there is no "o" in the "L" columns. From 1997 onwards, AIDS-specific mortality decreased by a factor $\exp(-3.26) = 0.038$ and natural mortality by a factor $\exp(-1.48) = 0.23$. The parameters in rows 8 to 11 quantify the additional effect of the combination of HCV and cART, the interaction term. After 1997, the effect of HCV coinfection on liver related mortality was a factor $\exp(-1.17) = 0.31$ lower than before 1997. For AIDS and natural COD, the effects of HCV coinfection were significantly increased compared to the pre-cART period.

For the effect of HCV coinfection within the cART period itself, we combine parameters. For liver related mortality, we add the parameter estimates in the rows 1 to 11 in the last "L" column that have an "o", and subtract the parameter estimates in the rows 1 to 11 in the third "L" column that have an "o" (which are absent). Hence we obtain RH $= \exp(3.48 - 1.17) = 10.1$. For the effect of HCV coinfection on the other CODs in the cART period, the "cART" effect in rows 5 to 7 cancels. For example, HCV coinfection increased AIDS related mortality by a factor $\exp(-0.45 - 3.26 + 1.48 + 3.26) = 2.80$. This is a factor $\exp(1.48) = 4.39$ stronger than the effect $\exp(-0.45) = 0.64$ of HCV coinfection on AIDS related mortality in the pre-cART period.

Effects of gender

In correspondence with the analysis of overall mortality (Figure 4.5), we assume that the effect of gender on mortality does not depend on HCV status. In the pre-cART period, we force the gender effect to be the same for every COD (parameter 12)[12]. Females had a lower mortality: RH $= \exp(-0.44) = 0.64$. Since females tend to be more adherent to cART, we allow the change in AIDS

---

[11]We assume HCV infection to have occurred before HIV infection. For IDU and persons with haemophilia, this is a reasonable assumption because HCV is highly infectious via blood. In MSM, HCV is transmitted sexually and infection mostly occurred at or after HIV infection. As a consequence, liver related mortality is likely to occur longer after HIV infection in MSM. However, since follow-up in HCV infected MSM was of limited duration and there were no liver related deaths observed, a separate parameter could not be estimated reliably.

[12]The numbers in Figure 4.6 suggest that the effect of HCV infection on non-natural mortality is increased in women before 97. Because of few deaths in women, we do not model a separate effect.

specific mortality after 1996 to depend on gender (parameter 14). For natural and non-natural mortality, we model a change for reasons that are explained in Chapter 5, but we require the size of the relative hazard to be the same for both. No effect is seen for either of the two (RH = exp(0.01) = 1.01). We don't allow for a change in liver related mortality after 1996, because we do the same for HCV negative males and we assume the effect of gender on liver related mortality not to depend on HCV status. Since all MSM are male, the gender effects only apply to the other three risk groups.

Effects of risk group

We assume liver related mortality to be equal for MSM, MSW and persons with haemophilia of the same age, gender and HCV status and with follow-up in the same calendar period. For the other CODs we assume this to hold for HIV mono-infected individuals only. In HCV coinfected individuals, we allow mortality in MSW and persons with haemophilia to differ from MSM, but assume the same relative effect over all CODs (parameter 15)[13].

IDUs may have a different spectrum of mortality due to their different lifestyle. For HIV mono-infected IDU in the pre-cART era, each of AIDS related (parameter 16), natural (17) and non-natural (18) mortality are allowed to differ from the other risk groups. HIV mono-infected IDU had a much higher non-natural mortality (RH = exp(2.34) = 10.4), but natural mortality and AIDS related mortality are not significantly increased.

We expect the change in AIDS related mortality in the cART era to be smaller than in the other risk groups because IDUs are less often successfully treated for HIV infection. Indeed, the relative hazard of exp(−3.26 + 0.48) = 0.062 is slightly larger, but the relative change exp(0.48) = 1.62 is not significant (parameter 19). For natural and non-natural mortality, we assume the change to be equal for both CODs (parameter 20). The value exp(−0.52) = 0.59 is again not significant.

We allow the effect of HCV infection in IDUs to be different from the other risk groups. We assume this effect to be the same for liver related, AIDS related and natural mortality (parameter 21). This value is not significant: RH = exp(0.26) = 1.30. It is believed that higher risk taking behaviour in HCV positive IDUs causes especially non-natural mortality to differ from other risk groups, but no such effect is found (parameter 22).

Effects of age

The effect of age on overall mortality was assumed to be independent of calendar period. Therefore, we assume the same for cause-specific mortality.

Mortality rate increases with increasing age, except for non-natural mortality. Therefore, for HIV mono-infected individuals, the effect of age is assumed to be equal for AIDS related, liver related and natural mortality. Indeed,

---

[13]We have no specific reason to expect a difference.

a strong age effect is seen (RH = exp(0.41) = 1.51 per 10 years increase in age at infection). For non-natural mortality the effect is weaker (RH = exp(0.25) = 1.28 per 10 years increase in age at infection).

We choose time since HIV infection as the principal time scale. For liver related mortality in HCV infected individuals, age may be a proxy for time since HCV infection. Therefore, we modeled a separate age effect (parameter 26). Indeed, the age effect on liver related mortality was exp(0.36) = 1.43 times stronger in HCV coinfected individuals, leading to a total increase in liver related mortality of exp(0.41 + 0.36) = 2.16 per 10 years increase in age. For the other CODs, we allow the age effect to differ from HIV mono-infected individuals as well, but assume this change to be equal for all three CODs (parameter 25). There is no indication of an additional age effect.

4.7 Summary

When estimating effects on the cause-specific or transition hazard, individuals leave the risk set when they experience a competing event. This is the same as what happens in a classical survival setting with a single event type. Therefore, we can use all the techniques and programs from classical survival analysis. What differs is the interpretation. Effects are not quantified on the marginal hazard but on the cause-specific/transition hazard. Only if the competing risks happen to be independent, then we also obtain effects on the marginal hazard. Although still generating confusion, these observations were already made 40 years ago [79].

By combining the data that is used in the analyses per event type into a stacked data set, the partial likelihood structure of the separate analyses is retained and all parameter estimates are obtained in one go. As a bonus, we obtain increased flexibility in modeling the effect of covariables [69]:

1. We can *test* whether the effect of a covariable differs between transitions. This may provide insights into disease mechanisms.

2. We can fit a model in which we *assume* that the effect of a covariable is equal for different transitions. Although the effect is unlikely to be exactly the same, it can be useful for reasons of parsimony. If a transition is rare, it may be necessary to make this assumption.

3. We can fit a model in which we assume a covariable to affect some of the transitions only. Again, this can be useful for reasons of parsimony.

4. We can assume proportional baseline hazards. This is useful if we want to quantify relative progression rates for different transitions via simple parameters.

In the combined analysis with the stacked data set, type-specific covariables can be created to obtain parameter estimates that have the same interpretation as in the analyses per event type. If we want to make more restrictive assumptions, we need to give careful attention to the choice of contrasts and their resulting interpretation.

Although attractive for its simplicity with respect to estimation, a drawback of a regression model for the transition hazard is that effects do not translate to similar effects on the risk. In Chapter 5, we explain why this happens and describe two alternative approaches to quantifying effects on the cumulative scale.

4.8 Exercises

1. In patients that receive allogeneic hematopoietic stem cell transplantation, relapse and treatment related mortality (TRM) are two competing events. Comment on the following statements:

> I. The effect of a covariable on an event from either a cause-specific (e.g. relapse) model or overall (e.g. relapse and TRM combined) model may be very different from the effect of the covariable on the event (e.g. relapse) in the presence of competing risks.

> II. Using a cause-specific Cox regression model is incorrect because it ignores competing risks and treats them as censored.

2. Sometimes we want to model effects of covariables that only have a meaning in a subgroup. For example, in Section 4.5.4 we quantified how the time of AIDS diagnosis influences the progression to death. Several rows referred to events before AIDS. We said that it was sufficient to assign the value zero—or any other constant value—to these rows. In this exercise we investigate this in more detail for a different setting.

Suppose we want to quantify the effect of pregnancy and age at first pregnancy on the risk of breast cancer before the age of 60. In Table 4.11 we show data from three women. Y is the dependent variable that tells whether the woman developed breast cancer before the age of 60. X_3 is a third covariable that gives information on the presence of a mutation

TABLE 4.11

Age at first pregancy; three example individuals

X_1: pregnant	X_2: age 1st pregnancy	X_3: BRCA1	Y: cancer
No	...	yes	yes
Yes	20	yes	no
Yes	35	no	yes

in the breast cancer susceptibility gene BRCA1. Women that have never been pregnant do not have a value for age at first pregnancy.

(a) What value would you fill in at the location of the three dots?

(b) Write down the logistic regression model that quantifies P(cancer) as function of X_1, X_2 and X_3; age at first pregnancy is modeled as a linear effect.

(c) Express the odds ratio of breast cancer via the parameters of the model for the following combinations

   i. women who first become pregnant at the age of 20 versus women who have never been pregnant

   ii. women who first become pregnant at the age of 35 versus women who first become pregnant at the age of 20

   iii. women who first become pregnant at the age of 35 versus women who have never been pregnant

(d) Suppose we had assigned the value 5.00 instead of 0.00 in column **aids.time** in Table 4.10. What would happen with respect to the parameter estimates in `fit.aidssi.mst4` on Page 166?

3. In the situation as described in Section 4.5.4, suppose that we allow the effect of `aids.time` to be different for transitions 4 (AIDS → death) and 6 (SI → death). In what way would the data in Table 4.10 need to change?

4. We formulate some questions based on the example in Section 4.6:

(a) On Page 174 we wrote "After 1997, the effect of HCV coinfection on liver related mortality was a factor $\exp(-1.17) = 0.31$ lower than before 1997". What does this mean? How large are the estimated relative hazards for both calendar periods?

(b) In Figure 4.7, we assume that parameter 19 contributes to the $\geq$ 97, HCV− group and $\geq$ 97, HCV+ group in the same way. How do you translate this into words?

Use Figure 4.7 to obtain the estimates for the following relative hazards:

(c) the effect of HCV coinfection on liver related mortality in male IDUs aged 30 in the pre-cART era

(d) the effect of HCV coinfection on liver related mortality in male IDUs aged 30 in the cART era

(e) the effect of HCV coinfection on AIDS related mortality before 1997 in male IDUs aged 30

(f) the effect of HCV coinfection on AIDS related mortality after 1997 in female MSW aged 30

(g) the effect of HCV coinfection on AIDS related mortality after 1997 in female MSW aged 40

(h) for AIDS related mortality in the cART era in male, mono-infected IDUs aged 30, compared to the other risk groups of same gender, age and infection status

(i) for AIDS related mortality in the cART era in female, coinfected IDUs aged 30, compared to MSW of same gender, age and infection status

(j) for AIDS related mortality in the cART era, compared to the pre-cART era, in male coinfected IDU aged 30

4.9 Software

Since everything that has been explained in this chapter boils down to fitting a Cox proportional hazards model, standard statistical software for survival analysis can be used. For data with left truncation and for clock-forward multi-state models, the program needs to allow for late entry.

The creation of the stacked data set can be done in a program of choice. In R you can use the functions `crprep` and `msprep` from the `mstate` package. Use of these functions was explained in Sections 2.9.1.2 and 3.7.3.

In the competing risks setting, we can use either of the two functions. It is recommended to use the `crprep` function if we also want to fit a regression model on the subdistribution hazard (Section 5.3), because it creates a weighted data set that allows for estimating the subdistribution hazard. If we specify all event types in its **trans** argument, we create the stacked data set in which the **failcode** variable specifies the event types. In the regression model for the cause-specific hazard, an individual that experiences a competing event leaves the risk set. This is attained by only selecting the rows with `count` equal to 1. The data set `aiddsi.stack` from Section 4.3.1 can be obtained from `aidssi.w` that we created in Section 2.9.1.2 using

```
aidssi.stack <- subset(aidssi.w, count==1)
```

In both functions, the covariables are included via the **keep** argument. The `mstate` package has a special function `expand.covs` to add transition-specific covariables to the stacked data set. The main required arguments are the name of the stacked data set and the names of the variables for which we need transition-specific versions. In the `aidssi.stack` data set we create the type-specific covariables for `ccr5` via

```
aidssi.stack <- expand.covs(aidssi.stack, covs="ccr5")
```

They are named by appending a suffix to the original name of the variable. If the stacked data set is created via `crprep`, the values in the **failcode** column are appended. In `aidssi.stack` we obtain new columns named **ccr5.AIDS** and **ccr5.SI**. If the stacked data set is created via `msprep`, the transition numbers .1, .2, ..., .K are appended. For categorical variables we can also choose a long form that includes the names of the levels that are not the reference value (**ccr5WM.AIDS** etcetera). For this we specify `longnames=TRUE`. Note that `longnames=TRUE` is the default if the data set is created via `msprep`. We can also create the variables ourselves, and if we want to use other contrasts this is often more straightforward. In the file `ExampleCode.R` on the book's website we show the R code to create the variables **tr.AIDS**, **tr.prop** and **aids.time** that were used in Section 4.5.

4.10   Computer practicals

If you are only interested in the competing risks setting, you can skip the second part of the practicals. Some of the issues that are covered in the competing risks practicals return in the multi-state ones.

Competing risks analysis

We quantify the effect of the EBMT score on the cause-specific hazards for relapse and death-without-relapse.

1. **Separate analyses** Quantify the effect of the EBMT score on both events by fitting two separate cause-specific proportional hazards models, using the `ebmt1` data set. Does a higher value of EBMT risk score increase the cause-specific hazards? Are the effects of EBMT score comparable for both event types?

2. **Combined analysis** Repeat the analyses, but now by fitting one proportional cause-specific hazards model for both competing risks at once. You can use the stacked data set `Webmt1`, which was created via the `crprep` function in Section 2.10.

   Fit the model in three ways:
   1. By including an interaction between the EBMT score and the type of end point
   2. By creating a single compound variable that combines the EBMT risk score and the type of end point
   3. By creating type-specific covariables

   Do all approaches give the same estimates? If not, can you translate one output into the other? Compare the estimates with those from the separate analyses.

   Test whether the proportional hazards assumption is reasonable.

3. **Test for equality of effects** Test the null hypothesis that the hazard of medium risk, relative to low risk, is the same for both event types. And similarly for high risk, relative to low risk.

Perform the likelihood ratio test of the null hypothesis that the effect of both medium and high risk is the same for both event types.

Multi-state analysis

We additionally investigate the effect of the EBMT risk score on death after relapse. And we investigate whether the effect of relapse on death has changed over time.

4. **Create and inspect the stacked data set** Create the stacked data set that is needed for the analyses. Include the variables the EBMT score (`score`) and year of relapse (`yrel`). Store the stacked data set in an object named `msebmt`. Compare the data of the first two individuals with the information in the `ebmt1` data set.

   Count the number of transitions between the different states, using the `events` function. Do the numbers correspond with the number of competing events and the overall number of deaths if you make the summary yourself based on the data in `ebmt1`? What additional information does the `events` function provide?

5. **Create transition-specific covariables** Create the transition-specific covariables for the EBMT score and year of relapse using the `expand.covs` function. Don't add them to the `msebmt` object yet, but create a separate data set `msebmt.tmp` via

   ```
   msebmt.tmp <- expand.covs(msebmt, c("score","yrel"))
   ```

   Have a look at the resulting data set. Study the values of the transition-specific covariables in relation to the original covariables and the transitions.

   Create the transition-specific covariables using the short variable naming and add them to the `msebmt` object. Compare this with the previous naming. What does, for instance, `score2.3` represent?

   The effect of `yrel` is only relevant for transition 3; why? So as not to be tempted to use it for other transitions, we delete the others. A sophisticated way of doing this makes use of regular expressions[14]:

   ```
   msebmt <- msebmt[,-grep("yrel..[1-2]", names(msebmt))]
   ```

6. **General model** Use the transition-specific covariables to estimate the effect of the EBMT score on all transitions, allowing this effect to differ by transition.

   Compare the hazard ratios of `score` for transitions 1 and 2 with those of

---

[14] We could also select the columns, e.g. via `msebmt <- msebmt[,-c(17,18,20,21)]`

the competing risks analyses in practicals 1. and 2. of this section. What do you notice? Do you have an explanation?

This model could also be obtained by fitting separate Cox regression models for each transition. How would you do this? You don't have to perform the actual computations.

7. **Same hazard ratios?** Looking at the hazard ratios of the medium EBMT score across the different transitions, would you say they are similar? And what about the hazard ratios for a high EBMT score? Perform the likelihood ratio test to see whether the hazard ratios for both the medium and high score may be considered equal across the transitions.

8. **Proportional baseline hazards** Based on the likelihood ratio test result, we continue with a model in which the effect of the EBMT score is assumed to be equal across the transitions.

   In order to quantify how much the death rate changes after a relapse, we will now look at a model where the baseline transition hazards into death are assumed to be proportional. Thus, the transitions 2 and 3 are assumed to share a common baseline.

   Create a covariable `rel.surv` that allows you to fit a model in which the baseline hazards to death are proportional. Fit the model and have a look at the results. What does the hazard ratio of `rel.srv` imply? Have the hazard ratios of `score` (or their standard errors) changed compared to the model in which we had a separate baseline hazard per transition? Test whether proportionality for the baseline hazards to death is a reasonable assumption.

   Compare the estimate of the standard error with a robust sandwich-type estimate.

9. **Time trend in relapse?** Now we are ready to study whether the effect of a relapse on mortality has changed over time. We will start from the model in Exercise 8 that assumes proportional baseline hazards for the two transitions into death.

   For transition 3, `yrel` is of importance, but the rows that refer to transitions 1 and 2 have missing values. Rows with missing values are removed when fitting a Cox model, which is not what we want. How do you solve this problem?

   Add period of relapse to the model. What is your conclusion with regard to the effect of period of relapse? Has the hazard ratio of `rel.srv` changed? Has the *meaning* of this hazard ratio changed?

   What is the hazard ratio of the transition into death after relapse in 2000+ with respect to the transition into death without relapse? Does a relapse nowadays (after 2000) have a (statistically) significant impact on the transition rate to death?

5

Regression; Translation to Cumulative Scale

5.1 Introduction

In the previous chapter we explained regression on the cause-specific hazard and its multi-state equivalent the transition hazard. The hazard is an instantaneous quantity that can be used to study and understand etiology. For prediction, effects on the cumulative probability are of more interest.

In the classical survival setting, the effect of a variable on the hazard translates to a qualitatively similar effect on the cumulative probability—the direction of an effect on the cumulative probability can already be learned from its effect on the hazard. For example, the CCR5-Δ32 deletion decreases the marginal hazard of AIDS, i.e. the hazard of AIDS if other events do not prevent AIDS from occurring. As a consequence, individuals with the deletion have a lower probability to develop AIDS within a certain time span. In the competing risks setting, effects on the cumulative scale may differ from effects on the cause-specific hazard. The reason for this phenomenon is that the cause-specific cumulative incidence is determined by all cause-specific hazards, also those from the competing events. We show this by means of a simple example in Section 5.2.1. Therefore, alternative regression models have been suggested, models in which parameter estimates do have a direct interpretation on the cumulative scale. We describe two such models.

Each of the three approaches that we discuss can be seen as an extension to the regression setting of one of the representations of the nonparametric estimator of the cause-specific cumulative incidence.

The Aalen-Johansen form in (2.14) is determined by the nonparametric estimates of all cause-specific hazards. In Section 5.2.1 we replace them by estimates that are based on a regression model for the cause-specific hazards. In Section 5.2.2 we use the same approach in the multi-state setting to translate effects on the transition hazards to transition probabilities.

The product-limit form in (2.17) is based on the nonparametric estimate of the subdistribution hazard for that cause. In Section 5.3 we replace this estimate by one that is based on a proportional subdistribution hazards model (often called the Fine and Gray model). Although this hazard is not a rate in the classical sense (see also the discussion on Page 87), it is a useful quantity because it qualitatively reflects how covariables affect the cumulative probability via a same type of relation as in the classical survival setting. If we are only interested in the direction of the effects on the cumulative scale and not in the cumulative probabilities themselves, we can restrict our analyses to the hazard.

The ECDF-form in (2.19) is based on a nonparametric estimate of the cumulative event probability itself. At any time t an individual has either experienced one of K event types or is still event-free. We can quantify the effect of covariables on this polytomous outcome via a multinomial logistic regression model. In Section 5.4 we describe a model that extends this to the whole time range: the proportional odds model.

In all three approaches, calculation of the cause-specific cumulative incidence is easy as long as all covariables are time-fixed. If the value of a covariable changes over time, quantifying effects on the cumulative scale is more involved. If the time-varying covariables can be represented via states in a Markov model, we obtain an internal and relatively easy way to translate effects to the cumulative scale ([23]; see also Page 164). An alternative is to use a landmark approach [23, 24].

Otherwise, we can still start with a model for the cause-specific or transition hazard. Quantifying effects of a time-varying covariable on the transition hazard is straightforward via the counting process representation (see Section 1.8.5). However, when we want to translate effects to the cumulative scale, we need to take the change in the variable over time into account. The same issues apply that were explained on Pages 38 and 39 for the classical setting. For the subdistribution hazard, although it is an instantaneous quantity, it is already not straightforward how to quantify the impact of a time-varying covariable on the hazard itself. In Section 5.3.3 we give two possible approaches, each with a different interpretation. Since the proportional odds model quantifies effects directly on the cumulative scale, time-varying covariables cannot be incorporated.

5.2   From cause-specific/transition hazard to probability

We concentrate on cumulative probabilities that are based on a proportional hazards model. However, the same approach can be used for other types of regression models for the cause-specific or transition hazard. We first explain the competing risks setting.

5.2.1   Competing risks

When using the Cox proportional hazards model in the classical survival setting, we use Formula (1.31) to translate effects to the cumulative scale. In the competing risks setting, we use the relation $F_k(t) = \sum_{t_l \leq t} \overline{F}(t_l-)\lambda_k(t_l)$ in (2.5). Because the overall survival $\overline{F}$ is determined by all cause-specific hazards, we can only quantify effects on the cumulative scale after we have fitted a model for all event types.

As an example, we quantify the effect of the CCR5-Δ32 deletion on the SI-specific cumulative incidence, based on the proportional cause-specific hazards model from Section 4.3. We obtained parameter estimates $\widehat{\beta}_{\text{AIDS}}$ for the effect of the deletion on the AIDS-specific hazard $\widehat{\lambda}_{\text{AIDS}}$ and $\widehat{\beta}_{\text{SI}}$ for the effect on the SI-specific hazard $\widehat{\lambda}_{\text{SI}}$. From (2.3) we know that the cumulative overall hazard is the sum of the cumulative cause-specific hazards, which we need in

$$\widehat{\overline{F}}(t \mid \text{ccr5}) = \exp\{-\widehat{H}(t \mid \text{ccr5})\} \tag{5.1}$$

$$= \exp\left\{-\left[\widehat{\Lambda}_{\text{AIDS}}(t \mid \text{ccr5}) + \widehat{\Lambda}_{\text{SI}}(t \mid \text{ccr5})\right]\right\}. \tag{5.2}$$

We use this to obtain the estimate of the SI-specific cumulative incidence in

$$\widehat{F}_{\text{SI}}(t \mid \text{ccr5}) = \sum_{t_{(i)} \leq t} \widehat{\lambda}_{\text{SI}}(t_{(i)} \mid \text{ccr5}) \times \widehat{\overline{F}}(t_{(i)} - \mid \text{ccr5})$$

$$= \sum_{t_{(i)} \leq t} \widehat{\lambda}_{0,\text{SI}}(t_{(i)}) \exp(\widehat{\beta}_{\text{SI}}\text{ccr5}) \times \tag{5.3}$$

$$\exp\left\{-\left[\widehat{\Lambda}_{\text{AIDS}}(t_{(i)} - \mid \text{ccr5}) + \widehat{\Lambda}_{\text{SI}}(t_{(i)} - \mid \text{ccr5})\right]\right\}.$$

Finally, we rewrite

$$\widehat{\Lambda}_{\text{SI}}(t \mid \text{ccr5}) = \sum_{t_{(i)} \leq t} \widehat{\lambda}_{\text{SI}}(t_{(i)} \mid \text{ccr5})$$

$$= \sum_{t_{(i)} \leq t} \widehat{\lambda}_{0,\text{SI}}(t_{(i)} \mid \text{ccr5}) \exp(\widehat{\beta}_{\text{SI}}\text{ccr5})$$

$$= \widehat{\Lambda}_{0,\text{SI}}(t) \exp(\widehat{\beta}_{\text{SI}}\text{ccr5}). \tag{5.4}$$

For the baseline SI-specific hazard $\widehat{\Lambda}_{0,\text{SI}}$ we can use the Breslow estimate (1.30) from the standard Cox model. The same holds for $\widehat{\Lambda}_{\text{AIDS}}$.

In Figure 5.1, we plot the estimates and compare them with the nonparametric estimates. For the wild type (WW), the curves practically overlap. Curves differ slightly more in the WM group, but note that the WM group is much smaller. In the estimates based on the regression model, the CCR5-specific curves for one event type jump at the same time points because they share the baseline hazard. As a consequence, the jumps for the WM group are much smaller than in the nonparametric estimates.

The protective effect of the CCR5-Δ32 deletion on progression to AIDS is also present in the cumulative probability. For SI as end point, a phenomenon is observed that cannot happen in the classical situation without competing risks. In the estimates based on the regression model, initially the probability of SI appearance is lower for the persons with the deletion WM, but after 11

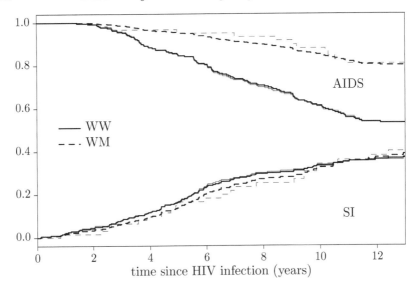

FIGURE 5.1
Cause-specific cumulative incidence for AIDS (on survival scale) and SI (on event scale). Grey: nonparametric estimate; black: estimate based on proportional cause-specific hazards model.

years the cause-specific cumulative incidence functions cross. Assuming proportionality in the cause-specific hazard does not translate to proportionality on the cumulative scale. Note that the cause-specific hazard ratio was 0.776 with a p-value of 0.29 (see Page 146), which is comparable to the p-value 0.28 of the log-rank test on the cause-specific hazards, but quite different from the p-value 0.94 of the log-rank test that compares the cause-specific cumulative incidences, i.e. the one based on the subdistribution hazards (see Table 2.4 on Page 84).

The reason for these results is that the protective effect of CCR5-Δ32 on the AIDS specific hazard is quite strong. This affects the effect of CCR5-Δ32 on the SI-specific cumulative incidence function.

We explain this by means of a simplified example in Figure 5.2. Suppose we have a population of 10,000 individuals with WW and 10,000 individuals with WM. We consider two time points, at which events of both types can occur. We assume that WW individuals have a constant event hazard of 30% at both time points, for both SI as well as AIDS. The CCR5-Δ32 deletion is protective for the SI-specific hazard (hazard ratio 26/30 = 0.87). However, it is even more protective for AIDS as a first event (hazard ratio 10/30 = 0.33). This latter aspect causes more WM individuals to remain at risk after the first event time (6400 versus 4000). As a consequence, at the next time point SI appears in

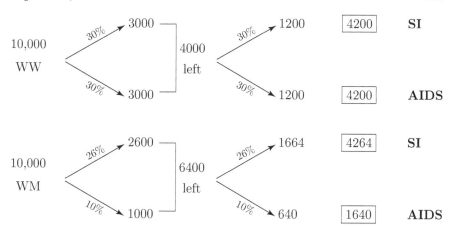

FIGURE 5.2
Explanation of the difference between effects on cause-specific hazard and on
cause-specific cumulative incidence.

more WM individuals than in WW individuals (1664 versus 1200). The total effect
after the second time point is that the cause-specific cumulative incidence for
SI appearance is higher for individuals with WM than for individuals with WW
genotype, 4264 versus 4200 individuals.

Note that not only the effect size itself, but also the baseline hazard determines whether the effect of a covariable on an event type affects the competing
cause-specific cumulative incidences. If a covariable has a large effect on an
event type that is relatively rare, it will have little impact on the competing
event types.

5.2.2 Multi-state models

In a multi-state setting, the basic idea is the same. The parameter estimates
for all transitions and the estimates of the cumulative baseline hazards are
plugged into the multi-state form of the Aalen-Johansen estimator (3.9). Only
the number of options increases [59], see also the list of considerations on
Page 111, and the computations become more tedious.

As an example, we compute transition probabilities based on the results
from the proportional transition hazards model of Section 4.5. We use model
fit.aidssi.mst3 (Page 163), in which we assumed the effect of age to be the
same for all transitions and in which we allowed the effect of the CCR5-Δ32
deletion to differ by transition, except for the transitions HIV $\rightarrow$ SI and AIDS
$\rightarrow$ AIDS/SI. We also assumed that the baseline hazards were proportional,
except for the transition HIV $\rightarrow$ AIDS.

We saw that, as long as the phenotype of the virus is NSI, individuals with the CCR5-Δ32 deletion have a much lower rate of progression to AIDS. For the other transitions, the effect of the CCR5-Δ32 deletion was not significant; one of the relative hazards was above 1 and all the others were below 1. Now we quantify the total effect on mortality.

For this, we calculate the fixed-history transition probabilities from the states HIV and SI to death for both values of CCR5. We choose two years as the starting time and we estimate $P_{04}(2,t)$ and $P_{24}(2,t)$ as function of time t. The estimates depend on all covariables in the model. If we quantify the effect of CCR5, we need to choose a reference value for age. Results are shown in Figure 5.3.

We see that, when the virus is of NSI phenotype, individuals with the CCR5-Δ32 deletion have a lower probability of dying within a certain time span than wild type individuals. If the virus has switched to SI phenotype, both death probabilities increase considerably and the advantage of having the CCR5-Δ32 deletion is smaller.

We can also quantify how the transition probability depends on age. Age is a continuous covariable, for which we choose a few values. In Figure 5.4 we plot the death risk for individuals aged 52 and individuals aged 27 that are wild type for CCR5[1]. The effect of age is seen from both the HIV state and the SI state. This is not surprising because we assumed the effect of age to be the same for all transition hazards.

If we wanted to show the effect of age over its whole range, we could add age as a another dimension. The extra dimension makes visualisation more difficult, although we could use a contourplot or a three-dimensional perspective plot. An alternative is to plot the estimates at a specific time point, e.g. ten years, and vary age.

5.3   Regression on subdistribution hazard

Similar to regression on the cause-specific hazard, it is common to assume the effects to be constant over time. This is the proportional subdistribution hazards model, which can be written as:

$$h_k(t \mid \mathbf{Z}_i) = h_{k,0}(t) \, \exp(\boldsymbol{\beta}_k^\top \mathbf{Z}_i) \,. \tag{5.5}$$

Parameters are estimated by maximizing a function that resembles the standard partial likelihood, but with the risk set adapted to estimation of the subdistribution hazard. In the estimator of the subdistribution hazard, individuals don't leave the risk set when they experience a competing event

---

[1]We use the values 25 and 50 years at HIV infection, but the estimates are calculated two years later.

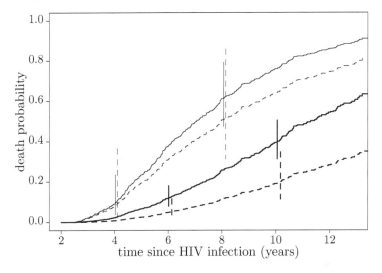

FIGURE 5.3
Transition probability from HIV (lower thick lines) and SI (upper thin lines) to death for `WW` individuals (solid lines) and `WM` individuals (dashed lines), aged 25 years at HIV infection. Error bars: 95% CI at specific time points.

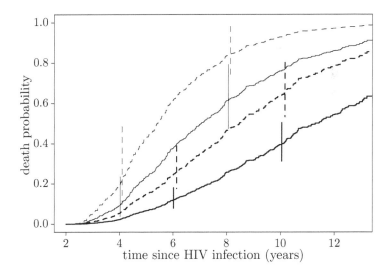

FIGURE 5.4
Transition probability from HIV (lower thick lines) and SI (upper thin lines) to death for individuals aged 27 years (solid lines) and 52 years (dashed lines) that have the wild type for CCR5. Error bars: 95% CI at specific time points.

(see Section 2.4). If there is no left truncation nor right censoring, individuals that experience a competing event remain in the risk set "forever" (see Section 2.4.1). If there is right censoring and we know when individuals would be censored if the competing event had not occurred, then one approach is to have them remain in the risk set until their potential censoring time. The general approach with left truncation due to late entry and/or right censoring is to use weighted at-risk sets that correct for this missed information. We use weights that are inspired by the nonparametric estimator of the subdistribution hazard in (2.26), but are now allowed to depend on covariables. For an individual l with covariable values $\mathbf{Z}_l$, we define an "at-risk" function as

$$\psi_l(t|\mathbf{Z}_l) = \begin{cases} \left\{ \widehat{\overline{\Gamma}}(t-|\mathbf{Z}_l)\,\widehat{\Phi}(t-|\mathbf{Z}_l) \right\}^{-1} & \text{if event-free and observed until } t \\ \left\{ \widehat{\overline{\Gamma}}(t_l-|\mathbf{Z}_l)\,\widehat{\Phi}(t_l-|\mathbf{Z}_l) \right\}^{-1} & \text{if competing event observed at } t_l < t \\ 0 & \text{otherwise} \end{cases}$$

(5.6)

$\widehat{\overline{\Gamma}}(t-|\mathbf{Z}_l)$ and $\widehat{\Phi}(t-|\mathbf{Z}_l)$ correct for the right censoring and left truncation respectively. We use the following weighted partial likelihood expression[2]:

$$L(\boldsymbol{\beta}_k) = \prod_{\substack{i=1 \\ e_i \delta_i = k}}^{N} \left\{ \frac{\psi_i(t_i|\mathbf{Z}_i)\exp(\boldsymbol{\beta}_k^\top \mathbf{Z}_i)}{\sum_{j=1}^{N} \psi_j(t_i|\mathbf{Z}_j)\exp(\boldsymbol{\beta}_k^\top \mathbf{Z}_j)} \right\}.$$

(5.7)

In order to find the $\boldsymbol{\beta}_k$ that maximize this function, we take the derivative to obtain the score function and set this to zero. If the truncation and censoring weights $\widehat{\Phi}$ and $\widehat{\overline{\Gamma}}$ are chosen to be the same for every individual, i.e. if they do not depend on covariables, this score function can be rewritten in a form based on the weights ω_l that were defined in (2.18). This estimating equation with ω-weights was originally proposed by Fine and Gray [34] for right censored data, and later extended to left truncated data [37].

The subdistribution hazard, being a hazard, is an instantaneous quantity. At the same time, because it is the hazard that corresponds to the cause-specific cumulative incidence, it qualitatively reflects effects on the cumulative scale via the relation (1.31). Hence, it provides an instantaneous approach to quantify effects on the cumulative scale. Contrary to the cause-specific hazard, we can restrict our analyses to one event type if it is the only one of interest. If all event types are of interest, we can perform all analyses at once if we first create a stacked data set, similar to what we explained in Chapter 4 for the cause-specific hazard.

There are three issues that need further discussion: how to choose the weight function, how to estimate the standard error and how to include time-varying covariables. Note that these are still partially open issues, on which research is ongoing. In the next three subsections, we give some ideas and suggestions.

---

[2]We assume that all event times of type k are distinct. In case of tied event times, we can use the Breslow or Efron approximation from the classical setting (see Page 38).

5.3.1   Choice of weight function

In Section 2.4 we assumed the subdistribution hazard to be the same for every individual. The product-limit estimator of the cause-specific cumulative incidence, which is based on the estimator of the subdistribution hazard, is equivalent to the Aalen-Johansen estimator if we choose the truncation and censoring weights to be the product-limit statistics from Section 2.4.2. This also holds if the distributions of entry time and/or censoring time depend on covariables; we can ignore this dependence as long as the same covariables do not impact the time of occurrence of any of the event types. If they do, then entry and/or censoring time are not independent of the event time distributions and we cannot use the standard nonparametric estimators.

One way to take account of covariables that affect the event time distribution is by quantifying their effects via a regression model, in casu the model for the subdistribution hazard. If the distributions of entry and censoring time do not depend on any of these covariables, we can use weights based on the product-limit statistics. Although no bias is introduced with this choice, it is not clear whether a more efficient estimator can be obtained if we make the truncation and censoring weights depend on covariables. In a simulation study, no difference was observed [92]. If the distributions of entry and censoring time do depend on one or more of the covariables in our regression model, we need to correct for it. If we consider only one categorical covariable Z, we can use a saturated model and calculate separate product-limit forms $\widehat{\Gamma}(t|Z)$ and $\widehat{\Phi}(t|Z)$ for every value of that variable. This was done in Section 2.9.2 to obtain Gray's log-rank test statistic. If we have a general regression model in which the subdistribution hazard depends on several covariables, which may be continuous as well as categorical, it is best to use $\widehat{\Gamma}(t|\mathbf{Z}_l)$ and $\widehat{\Phi}(t|\mathbf{Z}_l)$ that are based on some regression model as well. Fine and Gray suggested a Cox proportional hazards model [34], whereas Datta and Satten suggested to use Aalen's additive hazards model [27]. The optimal choice of the weight function is an ongoing research topic. The same issues play a role as when we use weights to correct for confounding due to imbalance in exposure groups or to correct for informative censoring (see Page 21).

If we allow the weights to depend on covariables, another open issue is whether we best use the weights $\psi_l(t|\mathbf{Z}_l)$, or the weights $\omega_l(t|\mathbf{Z}_l)$ that only affect individuals after they experienced a competing event. We based our partial likelihood specification in (5.7) on the ψ-weights, because this was how we derived the nonparametric estimator of the subdistribution hazard in (2.26). These same weights are the basis for estimation in the proportional odds model of Section 5.4. However, Fine and Gray suggest the use of ω-weights [34, p.500]. The weights $\omega_l(t|\mathbf{Z}_l)$ have the advantage that they lead to smaller data sets and the parameters can be estimated with standard software for fitting Cox models (see Section 5.7.2). As clarified in the next subsection, the uncertainty as quantified via the standard error may be obtained using the same standard software.

5.3.2 Estimation of standard error

Fine and Gray derived the asymptotic distribution of the parameter estimates when weights are used that do not depend on covariables [34]. Using the expression via ω-weights, they came up with a sandwich-type estimator of the standard error. In a simulation study, it was observed that the regular estimator of the standard error performed better in small samples [37]. The sandwich estimator of the variance tended to be too small, leading to confidence intervals that were too narrow. Although not investigated in the simulation study, the same is likely to hold if the ω-weights depend on covariables.

What could be the reason for the better performance of the regular estimator? Fine and Gray obtained a sandwich form of the standard error by rewriting $\widehat{\overline{\Gamma}} = \overline{\Gamma} + (\widehat{\overline{\Gamma}} - \overline{\Gamma})$; the second term gives rise to the sandwich form. $\widehat{\overline{\Gamma}}$ was seen as estimate of the true time-to-censoring distribution $\overline{\Gamma}$, suggesting that $\overline{\Gamma}$ is preferred over $\widehat{\overline{\Gamma}}$ as the weight function if it were known. However, using $\widehat{\overline{\Gamma}}$ is more efficient since it takes account of the random sampling variation. A similar phenomenon has been observed in casual inference: even if the theoretical exposure allocation mechanism were known, as in a randomized clinical trial, correcting for imbalance based on the data improves performance [105]. If $\overline{\Gamma}$ were the optimal weight and the sandwich standard error were needed to correct for the fact that $\overline{\Gamma}$ is estimated, we would expect the sandwich estimate to be larger on average than the regular one. However, in the simulation study it tended to be smaller. Another explanation for the better performance of the regular estimator may be that only individuals that do not experience the event of interest are reweighted in the ω-weights.

It is not clear which estimator performs better if the ψ-weights are used. In the proportional odds model in Section 5.4, estimation is based on the ψ-weights and a sandwich estimator of the standard error is more accurate.

5.3.3 Time-varying covariables

For estimation of the effect of time-varying covariables on the hazard, data is typically presented in the counting process format (see Section 1.8.5). Followup of an individual is split; a change in any of the covariables generates a new row. When estimating the subdistribution hazard, these rows can be used in two different ways, which impact the interpretation of the resulting estimates.

Pseudo-individual approach

One approach is to break the link with the original individual and interpret the rows as coming from different individuals. We call this the pseudo-individual approach. Each row represents a period during which the value of his covariables does not change. We can interpret the data set as having only time-fixed variables, in which each pseudo-individual has an "entry time", the start of the constant period, and a "censoring time", i.e. the end of the period, at which one of the covariables changes value again. These time points are included in the calculation of the truncation and censoring weights respectively.

As an example, we quantify the effect of the calendar period of follow-up on the spectrum of causes of death in HIV infected individuals (Section 5.3.4). For the first period we only use data until 1997 and we obtain censoring weights by terminating the follow-up of event-free individuals when they enter the second period[3]. For the second period, we only use follow-up after 1997. Individuals that contribute to both periods have the start of the second period as entry time. These entry times are included in the calculation of the truncation weights. We could say that for the first period we do as if we lived in 1997, whereas for the second period we do as if we started follow-up in 1997.

If calendar period were the only covariable, we could compute the nonparametric estimates for each period separately. This is how the estimates of the cause-specific cumulative incidence in Figure 4.4 were obtained. This approach is basically the same as when we estimate the hazard and product-limit Kaplan-Meier for both calendar periods separately in the classical survival setting with a single event type, for example if we looked at overall mortality as combined end point. Individuals that are event-free at the end of the first period contribute to the second period with a late entry.

If individuals that became HIV infected in the first period enter the second period, they are assumed to have the same hazard as the individuals that became infected in the second period. In the classical survival setting, there is only one event type and one hazard. However, the Kaplan-Meier only quantifies survival for the individuals that became infected in the second period. The disturbing effect of the first period makes the cumulative estimate not to represent the individuals that contribute to both periods. In the competing risks setting there are two possible hazards. In the pseudo-individual approach, when individuals that became infected in the first period enter the second period, they are assumed to be comparable to individuals that became infected after 1997 with respect to the cause-specific hazards. If all covariables are time-fixed, we use $\lambda_k(t) \times \overline{F}(t-) = h_k(t) \times \overline{F_k}(t-)$ (relation (2.12)) to derive that the subdistribution hazards are equal as well. This no longer holds if there are time-varying covariables. For individuals that contribute to both periods, the effect of the first period on the competing events impacts the cumulative probability. Although we align time-varying covariables with respect to the cause-specific hazard, we quantify their impact on the subdistribution hazard. This estimator of the subdistribution hazard is only valid for individuals that became HIV infected after 1997, for whom the time-varying covariable did not change value. Note that we could also restrict the analysis to the individuals that became infected after 1997. By including the individuals that became infected before 1997 and remained event-free and in follow-up until 1997, we increase the sample size for the second period.

---

[3]If there are no individuals lost to follow-up during the first period, an alternative is to use the end of the first period as administrative censoring time for the individuals that experienced a competing event.

In principle, the same pseudo-individual approach can be used to quantify the effect of an arbitrary time-varying covariable on the subdistribution hazard. To our knowledge, no such analyses have been performed yet, and the interpretation of the estimates thus obtained needs to be established.

Internal approach

The other approach is to interpret the rows as continuing follow-up from the same individual. We call this the internal approach, in analogy to the term internal left truncation [6]. The truncation weights are only determined by the entry times of the individuals, and the censoring weights are only determined by the censoring times of individuals that do not have any of the competing events observed during follow-up.

The internal approach has been used to investigate mortality and discharge as competing events in an intensive care unit [29]. In this study, follow-up was complete during the first 28 weeks—there were no late entries nor censored events. Therefore, the authors could estimate the subdistribution hazard until week 28 by having individuals that were discharged remain in the risk set with a weight of one. They considered one internal time-varying covariable: the sequential organ failure assessment (SOFA) score. They jointly modeled the development of SOFA score via a random effects model and the effect of SOFA score on mortality via a proportional subdistribution hazards model. For the SOFA score they used the fitted values from the random effects model.

In the analysis, individuals remain in the risk set after the competing event, but what value of SOFA score do we use? The SOFA score was only measured *until* the competing event. After non-lethal competing events like discharge, SOFA score values do exist. The authors predicted these values based on the joint model. However, there is no guarantee that the true values of the SOFA score after discharge are the same as the predicted ones that are based on a model of its development while an individual is event-free. If discharge is the event of interest and death is the competing event, values of the internal time-varying covariable do not even exist and are highly speculative. An alternative approach that has been suggested is to carry forward the value when the competing event occurred [11].

The authors evaluated their method via a simulation study. They assumed a model for the development of the SOFA score over the whole time range, also after the occurrence of the competing event. Parameter estimates were almost unbiased if the sample size was large enough. However, the SOFA score after the competing event was predicted based on the same model that generated the data, which is a highly idealized setting.

There are situations in which we know the value of a time-varying covariable after the occurrence of a competing event. One example is when the competing event is not observed and follow-up continues, such as with a cure as competing event in patients that are treated for cancer (see Page 88). Another example is when the time-varying covariable is external. In the study of causes of death in HIV infected individuals, Section 5.3.4, calendar period of (potential) follow-up is also known after an individual has died. In the internal approach, individuals that were infected and experienced a competing COD before 1997 are included in the risk set for the second period from 1997 onwards.

If we have randomly left truncated and right censored data, the values of the time-varying covariables are also needed in the calculation of the weights. In the weights $\psi_l(t|\mathbf{Z}_l(t))$, these values only need to be computed while an individual is observed to be in follow-up. In the weights $\omega_l(t|\mathbf{Z}_l(t))$, we also need the values after the competing event has occurred.

In the internal approach, we align time-varying covariables with respect to the subdistribution hazard; we do not assume that the cause-specific hazards are equal. In the study of causes of death in HIV infected individuals, we assume that the individuals that became infected before 1997 have the same subdistribution hazard $h_k(t)$ after 1997 as the individuals that became infected after 1997. If this is a valid assumption, we can use the estimates from the proportional subdistribution hazards model to quantify the cause-specific cumulative incidence after any date of HIV infection, whether it be before or after 1997.

5.3.4 Examples

We repeat the analyses from Sections 4.3 and 4.6, but now for the subdistribution hazard.

Impact of CCR5-Δ32 deletion on AIDS and SI switch

We use the combined analysis for both event types together, using the stacked data in `aidssi.stack`. Since we only have one dichotomous covariable, there are two straightforward choices for the weight function to correct for censored observations (there was no late entry): we can use the overall product-limit statistic or the product-limit statistic stratified by CCR5 value. If we use one overall product-limit statistic in the ω-weight function we obtain:

```
                   coef exp(coef) se(coef)     z     p
ccr.combWM.AIDS -1.0044     0.366    0.306 -3.28 0.001
ccr.combWM.SI    0.0236     1.024    0.236  0.10 0.920

Likelihood ratio test=13.9  on 2 df, p=0.000935  n= 5004,
                                    number of events= 220
```

We see that the CCR5-Δ32 deletion lowers the subdistribution hazard for AIDS by a factor 0.366. The relative hazard is slightly closer to one than the relative cause-specific hazard, which was 0.291^4. The protective effect on the deletion on AIDS impacts the cause-specific cumulative incidence to SI: the relative subdistribution hazard is 1.024, whereas it was 0.776 for the cause-specific hazard. The p-value of 0.92 is close to the p-value from the log-rank test for the null hypothesis that the SI-specific cumulative incidence curves are equal, which is basically a test for subdistribution hazards (Table 2.4 on Page 84). Note that both hazard models yield standard errors of comparable width. If we use the CCR5-specific weight function and the ω-weights, results are almost the same:

```
                coef exp(coef) se(coef)    z     p
ccr.combWM.AIDS -1.035    0.355    0.307 -3.38 0.001
ccr.combWM.SI    0.020    1.020    0.236  0.08 0.932


Likelihood ratio test=14.8  on 2 df, p=0.000604  n= 3850,
                                     number of events= 220
```

In Figure 5.5, we compare the predicted cause-specific cumulative incidence based on our model with the nonparametric estimates. The curves based on the regression model for the subdistribution hazard cannot cross. For SI, this is different from what we observe for the nonparametric estimates, and also for the estimates based on the regression model for the cause-specific hazard (Figure 5.1).

We can test whether the effect of the CCR5-Δ32 deletion is proportional on the subdistribution hazard via the scaled Schoenfeld residuals (see Page 39). When performing the test, an issue is whether it should be based on a sandwich estimator of the variance [112]. Using the sandwich estimator, the p-values when testing against a linear time trend are 0.196 for AIDS and 0.097 for SI. If we use the regular estimator, p-values are slightly smaller (0.140 for AIDS and 0.068 for SI). In an unpublished simulation study, we found that p-values based on the regular estimator tended to be larger. The type 1 error probability was closer to the true significance level. If the effect was not proportional, the sandwich estimator performed better with respect to power; the probability to reject the null hypothesis, the type 2 error, was larger than with the regular estimator. Further research is needed to determine which method is preferred.

Causes of death in HIV infected individuals

In Section 4.6 we quantified the effect of HCV coinfection and calendar period of follow-up on the death-specific hazards for four causes of death (COD). In a regression model on the cause-specific hazard, we corrected for the possible confounders gender, risk group and age. Calendar period of follow-up was included as a time-varying covariable.

---

[4]From relation (2.12) we derive that the subdistribution hazard itself is always smaller than the cause-specific hazard. The relative subdistribution hazard can be further away from one if the effect of the covariable is in opposite directions for competing event types.

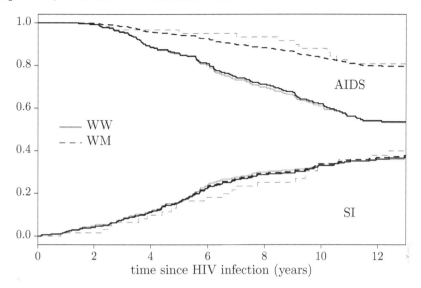

FIGURE 5.5

Cause-specific cumulative incidence for AIDS (on survival scale) and SI (on event scale). Grey: nonparametric estimate; black: estimate based on proportional subdistribution hazards model.

The cause-specific hazard quantifies the death rate among individuals that are alive. The introduction of cART has led to a large reduction in AIDS related mortality. Even if cART itself did not have an impact on other CODs, other CODs may be observed more frequently after 1997 because HIV infected individuals are much less likely to die of AIDS. We investigate this by means of a proportional subdistribution hazards model. We use the same analysis as was published in [104]. We model the effect of calendar period via the pseudo-individual approach, assuming calendar period to be aligned with respect to the cause-specific hazards. Hence, for the second period we quantify the impact of calendar period on the spectrum of CODs for individuals that became HIV infected after 1997. The weights due to late entry are based on the product-limit form per calendar period; we do not correct for any of the other variables. For the censoring weights $\widehat{\Gamma}$, one overall product-limit statistic is used. These choices may be too restrictive; more flexible weight statistics need to be investigated.

In Figure 5.6 we compare the estimates and 95% confidence intervals of the effects on the cause-specific hazards and the subdistribution hazards. The sequence and interpretation of the parameters is the same as in Table 4.7. Similar to the previous example, most parameters are closer to zero for the subdistribution hazard, but differences with the cause-specific hazard are not

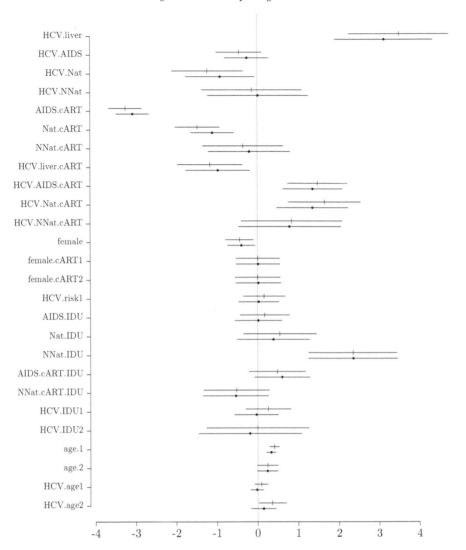

FIGURE 5.6
Effect estimates and 95% confidence intervals based on cause-specific hazards model (upper line) and subdistribution hazards model (lower line).

very large. Although HCV coinfection greatly increases liver related mortality, the effect on the subdistribution hazard for the other CODs is small. This may be explained by the fact that liver related mortality is rare. The large decrease in AIDS related mortality after 1997 has not caused other CODs to be observed much more frequently: all relative subdistribution hazards are still below zero for the reference group MSM aged 30.

5.4 Multinomial regression

At one specific time point t, either one of the competing events has happened, or an individual is still event-free. We specify a model on the odds of the occurrence of each of the event types, relative to being event-free, i.e.

$$\pi_k(t \mid \mathbf{Z}_i) = \frac{\mathrm{P}(T \le t, E = k \mid \mathbf{Z}_i)}{1 - \mathrm{P}(T \le t \mid \mathbf{Z}_i)}. \tag{5.8}$$

It extends the classical survival situation in which, at time t, the event status is dichotomous: the event has happened already $(T \le t)$ or is still to happen $(T > t)$. Then we specify a model on

$$\frac{\mathrm{P}(T \le t \mid \mathbf{Z}_i)}{1 - \mathrm{P}(T \le t \mid \mathbf{Z}_i)}.$$

We regress (5.8) on covariables via a multinomial logistic regression:

$$\log\{\pi_k(t \mid \mathbf{Z}_i)\} = \log\{\pi_{k,0}(t)\} + \boldsymbol{\beta}_k^\top \mathbf{Z}_i.$$

$\pi_{k,0}(t)$ is the intercept. We write it as function of t because we extend this structure over the whole time range. Since the effect of the covariables is assumed constant over time on the scale of the odds, it is called the proportional odds model. The effect of time itself is represented by the baseline odds $\pi_{k,0}(t)$. The proportional odds model has been extended to the multi-state setting [91].

Based on this model, the cause-specific cumulative incidence is

$$\mathrm{P}(T \le t, E = k \mid \mathbf{Z}_i) = \frac{\pi_{k,0}(t)\exp(\boldsymbol{\beta}_k^\top \mathbf{Z}_i)}{1 + \sum_{e=1}^{K} \pi_{e,0}(t)\exp(\boldsymbol{\beta}_e^\top \mathbf{Z}_i)}.$$

In the presence of left truncated and right censored data, parameters can be estimated via a maximum likelihood method in which individuals are weighted according to the at-risk function $\psi_l(t|\mathbf{Z}_l)$ in (5.6). For right censored data this has been investigated in [92, 20]. Based on results from a simulation study, it was concluded that more efficient estimates are obtained if weights are used that depend on $\mathbf{Z}_l$, even if the distribution of the censoring time does not depend on any of those covariables [92]. This was observed to be different from the regression model on the subdistribution hazard. The authors also observed that, contrary to the model for the subdistribution hazard, a sandwich estimator of the standard error clearly outperforms the regular estimator.

As an example, we estimate the effect of the CCR5-Δ32 deletion on the cumulative incidence for both event types. As parameter estimates we obtain $\widehat{\beta}_{\mathrm{AIDS}} = -1.39$ (p-value < 0.001) and $\widehat{\beta}_{\mathrm{SI}} = -0.174$ (p-value $= 0.565$). Hence, the conclusions are not different from the other two approaches. In Figure 5.7 the effects on the cause-specific cumulative incidence are shown. Similar to the proportional subdistribution hazards model, the proportional odds model does not follow the nonparametric estimate with respect to the crossing of the curves for SI as an event type.

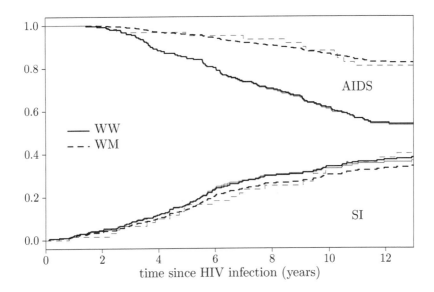

FIGURE 5.7
Cause-specific cumulative incidence for AIDS (on survival scale) and SI (on event scale). Grey: nonparametric estimate; black: estimate based on proportional odds model.

5.5 Summary

We quantified the effect of time-fixed covariables on the cumulative scale in three different ways. The first approach is based on methods from multi-state models. It is easy to fit the regression model on the cause-specific/transition hazard, but the translation of effects to the cumulative scale is somewhat involved. Since there is no one-to-one relation, it is not possible to summarize effects via a number of parameters. We need to quantify the effect for every possible combination of covariables. This makes this approach awkward for summarizing effects on the cumulative scale at the population level. However, it is not a problem if we only want to obtain an estimate for one specific combination of covariables, as is typically the case with individual prediction in a clinical setting. The second approach is to specify a regression model for the subdistribution hazard. It has become very popular in the competing risks setting. Sometimes it is even considered to be the only correct approach, which is certainly not true. The third approach is the proportional odds model, which directly quantifies the impact of covariables on the cause-specific cumulative incidence. It has not been used very often, which may be due to the availability of software.

In the proportional subdistribution hazards and the proportional odds model, parameters are typically estimated using inverse probability weights. An alternative approach has been suggested that is based on the use of pseudovalues [57]. Parameter estimates directly translate to similar effects on the cause-specific cumulative incidence. Therefore, if we are only interested in the direction of the effects on the cumulative scale, not in the prebabilities per se, we can restrict to fitting the model and report these parameter estimates. Apart from ease of use and interpretation of parameters, another argument used to choose a certain approach is the correctness of the model. All three models that we described assume proportionality of effects, each on a different quantity. In theory, only one of the three can hold for a specific study hypothesis and data set. In reality, proportionality will never be 100% correct, but if effects are much closer to proportional for one scale than for the others, that model may be the preferred choice.

Both the proportional hazards model and the proportional odds model can be seen as special cases of a general class of semi-parametric transformation models of the form [33, 36]

$$g\{F_k(t|\mathbf{Z}_i)\} = h_k(t) + \boldsymbol{\beta}_k^\top \mathbf{Z}_i . \tag{5.9}$$

These models specify the effect of the covariables over the whole time range, but assume that the effect of time on the scale of the link function g does not depend on the covariables. If $g(x) = \log\{-\log(1-x)\}$, we obtain the proportional subdistribution hazards model with $h_k(t)$ the logarithm of the integrated baseline hazard. With $g(x) = \log\{x/(1-x)\}$, we obtain the proportional odds model. The additive model, which has $g(x) = x$ as link function, has been advocated as most natural in competing risks settings [56].

If some of the covariables vary over time, estimation becomes more involved. Quantifying effects on the cause-specific hazard itself is easy to perform and interpret. For the subdistribution hazard, estimation and interpretation are less straightforward because individuals remain in the risk set after they have experienced a competing event. If we want to translate effects to the cumulative scale and a covariable changes as a consequence of the internal process that leads to the end point, we additionally need to model its development.

The approaches explained in this chapter can be used to obtain predictions at the cumulative scale, based on a regression model. We did not address the question how covariables in such models are selected. We refer to the general literature on prediction models [45, 97] and extensions to competing risk settings (e.g. [110, 109]).

In the Epilogue (Chapter 6), we return to the questions that were raised in Chapter 1: which quantity and what type of model is best used when answering a certain study question. Hopefully, by using the extra information that we provided in the previous chapters, you will now be better able to answer these questions for your own research.

5.6 Exercises

1. Suppose we have two competing event types, say 1 and 2, and two groups, say I and II. Suppose the cause-1-specific hazard is equal in both groups, but the cause-2-specific hazard is larger in group I. What can we say with respect the relative size of the subdistribution hazards for cause 1?

2.* The theoretical counterpart of Equation (5.2) can be written as

$$\overline{F}(t \mid \text{ccr5}_i) = \exp\left\{-\Lambda_{\text{AIDS}}(t \mid \text{ccr5}_i)\right\} \times \exp\left\{-\Lambda_{\text{SI}}(t \mid \text{ccr5}_i)\right\} \quad (5.10)$$

Comment on the following statement

> Using the general relation $P(T > t) = \exp\{-\int_0^t h(s)ds\}$ between survival function and hazard (see (1.9)), the right-hand side is a product of the marginal distributions $P(T_{\text{AIDS}} > t \mid \text{ccr5}_i)$ and $P(T_{\text{SI}} > t \mid \text{ccr5}_i)$. Furthermore, its product structure defines independence:
>
> $$P(\min\{T_{\text{AIDS}}, T_{\text{SI}}\} > t) = P(T_{\text{AIDS}} > t) \times P(T_{\text{SI}} > t)$$
>
> Therefore, equations (5.10) and (5.2) only hold if the distributions of time to AIDS and time to SI are independent.

5.7 Software

5.7.1 From cause-specific/transition hazard to probability

In Stata, the command stcompadj translates results from a semiparametric proportional cause-specific/transition hazards model to cumulative probabilities. The command `stpm2` fits proportional hazards models in which the baseline hazard is a smooth parametric function of time. If the baseline hazard is modeled flexibly enough, results are similar to those from the semiparametric model. The `stpm2cif` command translates estimates to the cause-specific cumulative incidence [46], whereas the `stpm2illd` command does the same for the illness-death setting.

In SAS, estimates from a proportional cause-specific hazards model can be translated to the cause-specific cumulative incidence via the macros `CumInc.sas` and `CumIncV.sas`[5]. We do not know of an extension to the multistate setting.

In R, we can use the `mstate` package to translate estimates from a proportional cause-specific/transition hazards model to cumulative probabilities. The same functions apply that were explained in Section 3.7.3 for nonparametric estimation. The first step is to fit a proportional hazards model via the `coxph` function. Whereas in Section 3.7.3 we used `strata` on the right-hand side of the formula, we now specify a regression model for the cause-specific/transition hazard as was explained in Chapter 4. The second, most laborious step is to use the `msfit` function. We need to define the covariable combination for which we want the estimates. The third step, applying the `probtrans` function to translate the cumulative hazards to probabilities, is completely similar to what was explained in Section 3.7.3.

We explain how to specify the covariable combination in `msfit`. The structure of `msfit` is similar to that of the `survfit` function in the `survival` package, but tuned to its use in multi-state models. They can be sued to compute nonparametric estimates of the survival (`survfit`) and transition (`msfit`) probabilities. But they can also compute predictions based on the results from a proportional hazards model.

In the first argument of both functions we specify the fitted proportional cause-specific hazards model on which we want to base our predictions. The covariable combination for which we want the predictions is specified via the second argument, `newdata`. This combination should be given in the form of a data frame in which all the covariables that were used in the regression model are given a value. In `survfit`, we can obtain predictions for several individuals with different covariable combinations at once. Different rows represent individuals with different covariable combinations, unless we specify the `id` argument[6]. In `msfit` we can only specify one covariable combination at a time. We need to create a stacked data set in which there is a row for every possible transition. The row position in the data set should be according to the transition number. If the proportional hazards model contains a stratum variable, in `msfit` that variable should be named `strata`. The other arguments—`variance`, `vartype` and `trans`—were already explained in Sec-

---

[5]See http://staff.pubhealth.ku.dk/~pka
[6]See the help file of `survfit.coxph`.

tion 3.7.3. Note that only the Aalen estimator of the variance can be used in the regression setting.

Competing risks

We explain the code for the SI/AIDS example (Section 5.3.4). We use the model from Page 148:

```
fit.stacked <- coxph(Surv(time, status) ~ ccr.comb +
                          strata(failcode), data = aidssi.stack)
```

We use the function **trans.comprisk** to define the transition matrix in the competing risks setting. Its first argument specifies the number of competing end points. The optional second argument specifies the names of the states.

```
trans.SI <- trans.comprisk(2, c("event-free","AIDS","SI"))
```

gives as matrix

```
              to
from          event-free AIDS SI
  event-free          NA    1  2
  AIDS                NA   NA NA
  SI                  NA   NA NA
```

We want to compute the cause-specific cumulative incidence for both values of the CCR5 genotype. For each we create a separate data frame.

```
indiv.WW <- data.frame(strata=c("AIDS","SI"), ccr.comb="WW")
indiv.WM <- data.frame(strata=c("AIDS","SI"),
                          ccr.comb=c("WM.AIDS","WM.SI"))
```

If the model has many covariables, which all need to be given a value, an alternative way is to directly select an individual from the stacked data set whose covariables are equal to the values that we want. In our example the first and second individual already contain the values WW and WM. We only need to add the **strata** variable that has the same values as **failcode**[7]. Hence, an alternative way to create the new individuals is

```
indiv.WW <- subset(aidssi.stack, id==1)
indiv.WW$strata <- indiv.WW$failcode
indiv.WM <- subset(aidssi.stack, id==2)
indiv.WM$strata <- indiv.WM$failcode
```

Now we are ready to apply the **msfit** function:

```
Haz.WW <- msfit(fit.stacked, newdata=indiv.WW, trans=trans.SI)
Haz.WM <- msfit(fit.stacked, newdata=indiv.WM, trans=trans.SI)
```

---

[7]We could also rename the **failcode** column.

The structure of the resulting object was explained on Page 140. To obtain the estimate of the cause-specific cumulative incidence, we use the `probtrans` function:

```
AJprop.WW <- probtrans(Haz.WW, predt=0)
AJprop.WM <- probtrans(Haz.WM, predt=0)
```

We refer to Section 3.7.3 for the structure of the resulting object. In the competing risks setting, there is only one outgoing state. Therefore, all estimates are in the first component of the list that is the output of the `probtrans` function. For example, the curves in Figure 5.1 that are based on the proportional cause-specific hazards molde are added to the nonparametric estimates via

```
lines(pstate3~time, data=AJprop.WW[[1]], type="s")
lines(pstate3~time, data=AJprop.WM[[1]], type="s", lty=2)
lines(1-pstate2~time, data=AJprop.WW[[1]], type="s")
lines(1-pstate2~time, data=AJprop.WM[[1]], type="s", lty=2)
```

Multi-state

In the multi-state setting, predictions are obtained in the same way. We use the proportional hazards model that was fitted in Section 5.2.2:

```
fit.aidssi.mst3 <- coxph(Surv(Tstart,Tstop,status) ~
      strata(tr.AIDS) + tr.prop + I(age.inf/10) +
   ccr5.23 + ccr5.1 + ccr5.4 + ccr5.5 + ccr5.6, data=aidssi.mst)
```

Since there are six transitions in the model, the data set that is specified in the `newdata` argument of `msfit` has six rows. The row ordering follows the transition numbers as defined in the transition matrix `trans.mst` in Section 3.7.3. We predict for an individual aged 25 years at HIV infection and for both values of CCR5. For a wild type individual, all `ccr5` related variables have the value zero. For an individual with the CCR5-Δ32 deletion, a `ccr5` related variable has the value 1 if the transition it codes for coincides with the row number. Hence, such an individual is specified as

	age.inf	strata	tr.prop	ccr5.23	ccr5.1	ccr5.4	ccr5.5	ccr5.6
1	25	1	2	0	1	0	0	0
2	25	2	2	1	0	0	0	0
3	25	2	3	1	0	0	0	0
4	25	2	4	0	0	1	0	0
5	25	2	5	0	0	0	1	0
6	25	2	6	0	0	0	0	1

The R code to create this individual can be found in the file `ExampleCode.R` on the book's website. Often, the easiest approach is to define all variables. Selecting an individual with the required combination from the stacked data set, as we suggested in the competing risks example, is usually less convenient. The reason is that usually no individual has been at risk for all transitions.

An individual may not have been in later states because he was censored. And if he has reached an absorbing state, one pathway often excludes another.

Once the new data set has been created, the estimates are simple to obtain. For example, the curves in Figure 5.3 for the individual with the deletion are based on estimates that were obtained via

```
trHaz.WM25 <- msfit(fit.aidssi.mst3, newdata=patWM25,
                                     trans=trans.mst)
prob.WM25 <- probtrans(trHaz.WM25, predt=2)
```

5.7.2   Regression on subdistribution hazard

All options that are described in this section make use of the ω-weights[8].

There are a couple of programs that calculate the weights and fit the model in one go. In Stata from version 11 onwards, the `stcrreg` command can be used. The `stcurve` command can be used to plot the cause-specific cumulative incidence for a combination of covariables [44]. In SAS from version 9.4 onwards, the `PROC PHREG` procedure from SAS/STAT version 13.1 can be used. In R, we can use the `crr` function in the `cmprsk` package. The `FGR` function in the `riskRegression` package provides a formula interface to the `crr` function. Only censoring weights are computed; weights to correct for late entry are not incorporated. The weights are based on the product-limit statistic of the censoring times, possibly stratified by a categorical variable. All use the sandwich estimator of the standard error.

An alternative is to create the data set with time-varying weights ourselves. With this data set, the proportional subdistribution hazards model can be fitted using the standard procedure for fitting a Cox model, if it allows for the inclusion of probability weights. This approach offers a lot of extra flexibility. It looks like we can do anything that can be done in a classical Cox analysis, but now in the competing risks setting of the subdistribution hazard. We not only estimate the parameters, but also obtain a proper quantification of the uncertainty in the estimates (see Section 5.3.2). We can fit the effect of covariables on all event types at once using a stacked data format, we can test for proportionality using scaled Schoenfeld residuals, and we can predict the cause-specific cumulative incidence for a specific combination of covariables. Furthermore, if we want to fit several models then the weights need to be computed only once. This offers speed improvements relative to the options in the previous paragraph.

In Section 2.9.1.2 we mentioned procedures to create the weights in Stata (via `stcrprep`), in SAS (via `%PSHREG`) and in R (via `crprep`). The SAS macro by default fits the model in one go, but one can choose to only generate the data set; in Stata and R the Cox model is fitted as a second step. Only the

---

[8]As long as the weight function is chosen to be the same for every individual in the data set, the ψ-weights give the same likelihood specification.

Stata version currently allows the weight function to depend on covariables via a regression model.

We show how the model is fitted in R, using the CCR5 example. We use the `crprep` function and have the `ccr5` variable included in the data set via the `keep` argument (if we use one overall weight function) or the `strata` argument (if the weight function depends on the CCR5 value). In Section 2.9, the resulting data sets were called `aidssi.w` and `aidssi.wCCR` respectively.

We use the standard `coxph` function to fit the model, but specify probability weights. We obtain the results on Page 195 if we quantify the effect of the CCR5-Δ32 deletion on both event types at once via[9]

```
fit.FG <- coxph(Surv(Tstart,Tstop,status==failcode) ~ ccr.comb +
            strata(failcode), data=aidssi.w, weights=weight.cens)
```

After the model has been fitted, we can use the functions that have been written to digest and validate results from the `coxph` function. To obtain predictions on the cumulative scale, we create a data frame with all possible covariable combinations and use this in the `newdata` argument of the `survfit` function:

```
indivs <- data.frame(
            ccr.comb=factor(c("WW","WW","WM.AIDS","WM.SI")),
                    failcode=c("AIDS","SI","AIDS","SI"))
pred.sdh <- survfit(fit.FG, newdata=indivs)
```

If the model contains a stratum variable, `survfit` has two options. If the variable is named strata in the new data frame, then for each given covariable combination curves are computed for all values in `strata`. If we use the original column name, as we did above, then the curve is only computed for the specific combination of covariable values and stratum value as specified in that row. Hence, if we had called the second column `strata` instead of `failcode`, we would have obtained a data frame with eight rows instead of four.

We can use the selection function for the `survfit` output to summarize and plot the curves for a subset of the individuals. Since rows 2 and 4 in `newdata` contain the data for SI as end point, `pred.sdh[c(2,4)]` gives the estimates of the SI-specific cumulative incidences for both values of CCR5. In Figure 5.5, we first compute and plot the nonparametric estimates, after which the four curves based on the proportional subdistribution hazards model are added via

```
lines(pred.sdh[c(2,4)], mark.time=FALSE, fun="event", lty=1:2,
                                                        lwd=2)
lines(pred.sdh[c(1,3)], mark.time=FALSE,  lty=1:2, lwd=2)
```

We can test for proportionality of the subdistribution hazards against deviations of the form $\beta(t) = \beta + \theta g(t)$ via the `cox.zph` function. If we test against a linear trend, $g(t) = t$, we write

---

[9]We first need to create the `ccr.comb` variable, similar to what we did in Section 4.3

```
cox.zph(fit.FG, transform="identity")
```

and obtain

	rho	chisq	p
ccr.combWM.AIDS	0.100	2.18	0.1398
ccr.combWM.SI	0.121	3.20	0.0735
GLOBAL	NA	5.38	0.0678

The test that is based on the sandwich estimator of the standard error has been implemented in the psh.test function in the crrSC package [112].

5.7.3 Proportional odds model

The timereg package contains the function comp.risk[10]. comp.risk can fit regression models on the cause-specific cumulative incidence for several types of link functions as in (5.9). It extends this formula by also allowing for effects that change over time. As two special cases, it can fit proportional subdistribution hazards models (via the argument model="fg" or model="prop") and proportional odds models (via the argument model="logistic").

It only allows for right censored data. The type of weight function is chosen via the cens.model argument. The product limit statistic can be chosen (cens.model="KM", the default), but it can also be made to depend on covariables via a Cox regression model (cens.model="cox"). By default it removes the first 10 percent or 20 event times in the estimation[11]. Therefore, it is best to specify the event times of interest explicitly via the times argument. The function does not allow for missing values; they need to be removed first. It uses a function Event to specify the observed event time data structure. The cause argument specifies the cause of interest.

In the example from Section 5.7.3, a proportional odds model for SI as event of interest is fitted via

```
fit.Podds <- comp.risk(Event(time,status)~const(ccr5),
              data=subset(aidssi,!is.na(ccr5)), cause=2,
              times=subset(aidssi,!is.na(ccr5)&status==2)$time,
                                          model="logistic")
```

The model fit can be obtained via the summary function. If we only want the parameter estimates, we can ask for the coefficients via coef(fit.Podds) and obtain

	Coef.	SE	Robust SE	z	P-val
const(ccr5)WM	-0.174	0.303	0.303	-0.576	0.565

If we want the estimate of the cause-specific cumulative incidence based on the model, we use the predict.comprisk function. Its basic specification is

---

[10]It also contains the function prop.odds.subdist that we don't explain here.

[11]This is for numerical stability if we allow effects to change over time.

very similar to the `survfit` and `msfit` functions that have been explained before. The required covariable combination is first created as a data frame, which is supplied to the `newdata` argument.

For the proportional subdistribution hazards model, it uses an estimation approach that is different from the one suggested by Fine and Gray. In an unpublished simulation study with one dichotomous covariable, we found the `timereg` approach to yield estimates that were slightly less efficient.

5.8   Computer practicals

Competing risks analysis

We compute the cause-specific cumulative incidence of both relapse and death-before-relapse for each value of EBMT score. We use two models: the proportional cause-specific hazards and the proportional subdistribution hazards model. In both approaches, we allow the effect of EBMT score to differ by event type and we assume separate baseline hazards.

1. **From cause-specific to cumulative** Perform the calculations based on the model for the cause-specific hazards from Section 4.10. Make a graph that compares the predicted cause-specific cumulative incidence with the nonparametric estimates. Use the overlaid format for the three values of risk score and the separate format for the two event types. Do the estimates correspond?

2. **Effects on subdistribution hazards** Quantify the effect of EBMT score on the subdistribution hazards for both event types. Compare the parameter estimates with the ones from the proportional cause-specific hazards model. Can you explain the difference?

   Make a graph that compares the predicted cause-specific cumulative incidence with the nonparametric estimates. Use the overlaid format for the three values of risk score and the separate format for the two event types.

   Test whether the proportional hazards assumption is reasonable.

5.8.1   Multi-state analysis

In Section 4.10 we investigated the effect of EBMT score on the transition hazards. Now we quantify what happens with respect to the transition probabilities. We use the proportional transition hazards model that i) assumed the effect of EBMT score to be the same for all transitions, ii) included an effect of calendar period on the transition from relapse to death and iii) assumed the two transition hazards to death to be proportional.

3. **Cumulative transition hazards** Compute all three cumulative transition hazards for an individual with a low EBMT score. For the transition from relapse to death, assume that relapse occurred in the period 1993-1996. Assign the result to an object named HvH and have a look at its structure.

   Understand what is happening here:

   ```
   H0 <- HvH$Haz[HvH$Haz$trans==2,]
   H1 <- HvH$Haz[HvH$Haz$trans==3,]
   head(H1$Haz/H0$Haz)
   ```

   Make a plot of the three cumulative transition hazards in overlaid format.

4. **Impact of year of relapse on hazard** Make a graph with the cumulative transition hazards from relapse to death for each relapse period as well as the transition hazard directly from transplantation to death. Use the reference category for the EBMT score (i.e. low risk).

   Hint: If the result of the regression model has been stored in `fit`, you can use the following code

   ```
   H2 <- H3 <- H1
   H2$Haz <- H2$Haz*exp(coef(fit)[3])
   H3$Haz <- H3$Haz*exp(coef(fit)[4])
   ```

   Understand why. Can you think of an alternative way to obtain the results?

5. **Transition probabilities** The impact of the period of relapse on death looks quite impressive, but the question remains how large the impact is for a population followed from transplantation; after all, if hardly anyone gets a relapse, a large difference in mortality after relapse will not have a big impact on a population. In order to study this we need to compute the probability of dying after transplantation, with or without relapse, for the three different relapse periods.

   Compute the transition probabilities for an individual that had a low EBMT score and a relapse in 1996-1999. Make a graph that shows all state occupation probabilities for such an individual. Think about the best display format of the curves.

   What does a probability of death, starting from transplantation, mean for a patient with a relapse between 1993 and 1996?

6. **Impact of year of relapse on transition probability** Compare the transition probabilities for patients having a relapse in 1993-1996 with those obtained from patients having a relapse in 1997-1999, or 2000+ (and with the same EBMT risk score, low risk). What is your conclusion?

   Hint: In order to obtain these probabilities we repeat what we have just done, changing only the value of `yrel` where necessary in the new data set. The code is tedious, but straightforward.

Would you expect the impact of period of relapse on survival after transplant to be stronger for a high risk patient? Repeat what you have done for a patient with a high EBMT risk score.

6

Epilogue

6.1 Which type of quantity to choose?

The two main reasons to perform a statistical analysis in medicine and epidemiology are to unravel disease etiology and to obtain accurate predictions. The effect of a covariable is often quantified via the hazard or rate, which is an instantaneous quantity. For prediction, which concerns the future, the cumulative probability or risk is the quantity of interest. If there is only a single event type of interest, there is only one hazard, and effects on the hazard translate to qualitatively similar effects on the cumulative probability.

If there are competing event types, the situation is more complicated. Several instantaneous and cumulative quantities can be defined (see Table 1.1). With choice, there is confusion with respect to the appropriate quantity and the interpretation of the results. We summarize which quantity is best suited to answer a specific type of research question, and whether and how it can be estimated.

The best choice of quantity has been debated in several papers. A classical example is the discussion on how to study late complications of radiation therapy in patients with cancer. Caplan *et al.* [18] advised to use the cause-specific cumulative incidence, because it estimates the probability that a patient actually develops a late effect. The argument was criticized by Bentzen *et al.* [9]. They argued that individuals that receive a lower dose of radiation are more likely to die early, and therefore the smaller number of observed complications in the lower dose group may be explained by earlier removal from the risk set. For this reason, they advocated the use of the Kaplan-Meier. Chappell [21, 22] tried to reconcile both viewpoints and argued that the type of approach depends on the question of interest. A radiation oncologist is more interested in the causal effect of radiation dose on late complications, which is better quantified by the Kaplan-Meier. (We prefer a plot of the cumulative cause-specific hazard because the Kaplan-Meier analysis may falsely be interpreted as an estimate of the marginal distribution; see also the IDU-MSM comparison below.) A patient is more interested in the fact that a higher dose decreases his death risk, even though it may increase the probability that he will experience late complications. This is quantified by the cause-specific cumulative incidences for late complications and death. Basically the same distinction was suggested by Koller *et al.* [61]: etiology is best described by the cause-specific hazard, whereas for prediction a quantification of effects on the cumulative scale is preferred.

Etiology

We agree that etiology can be described by the cause-specific hazards if the competing risks are different end points of the same biological process. An example is the process of ageing and its effect on the spectrum of causes of mortality. We quantify the different cause-specific death rates amongst the individuals that are still alive, i.e. at risk. The marginal hazard is the quantity of interest if we want to describe the effect of ageing on one specific cause of death. If the causes of death are, at least partly, consequences of the same biological process, individuals that die of one cause are also more likely to die of other causes: time to the competing causes of death is dependent. As a consequence, individuals that die of a competing event are different from individuals that remain alive, and the cause-specific hazard is different from the marginal hazard. Often the marginal hazard is not easy to conceptualize, unless we are able to describe the process in so much detail that we have separate pathways for the different causes of death. Then the causes of death become conditionally independent.

If the competing risk is the consequence of an intervention, then etiology is often best described by the situation in which the intervention is absent, which is quantified by the marginal hazard or marginal risk. An example is discharge as intervention if staphylococcus infection in hospital is the event of interest: the marginal distribution describes what would be observed if everyone would stay in hospital. It reflects the etiology of infection as a consequence of food hygienic conditions. We may also be interested in the marginal distribution if the competing risks reflect biological processes that are not related to the event of interest. An example is the comparison of the natural progression to AIDS in IDUs and MSM (Example 1. in Section 1.2.2). The causes of death in Table 1.2 are a combination of "interventions" (violence, accident, overdose, suicide) and biological mechanisms (liver cirrhosis, heart attack, HIV related infections). Liver cirrhosis and heart attack are not related to HIV infection, but death from HIV related infections is. This is more an issue of definition: although these individuals never had a formal AIDS diagnosis, it is clear that they died as a consequence of HIV infection and it may be better to give them an AIDS diagnosis when they died.

We can estimate the marginal distribution in a simple way only if the censoring due to the competing risks is noninformative. Then, individuals that are censored because they experience a competing event can be represented by the ones that remain at risk, which allows us to interpret the estimate as the event rate for the situation in which the competing events did not exist. By censoring individuals at their competing event time, we not only obtain an estimate of the cause-specific hazard but also of the marginal hazard. Although the hazard estimate can be interpreted as cause-specific as well as marginal, the resulting estimates of the cumulative probabilities are different: for the net risk we use the Kaplan-Meier, for the crude risk we use the estimator that was explained in Chapter 2. For example, if staphylococcus infection in hospital and discharge are unrelated, we estimate both the cause-specific as well as the marginal hazard of infection if we censor individuals at discharge. If used in the Kaplan-Meier, we estimate the marginal distribution; if used in the Aalen-Johansen estimator, we estimate the infection-specific cumulative incidence.

Usually the competing risks are not independent. By censoring individuals when they experience a competing event, we only estimate the cause-specific hazard. Whether this estimate is close to the marginal hazard depends on when the event of interest would have happened if a competing event happened first. On one extreme, if it would have happened right after the competing event, then the marginal hazard is equal to the overall hazard that combines all event types. On the other extreme, if it would never have happened, then the marginal hazard is equal to the subdistribution hazard.

The effect of a covariable on marginal hazard and cause-specific hazard may even be in opposite directions. This can occur if individuals that have the higher marginal event risk are more likely to receive an intervention that reduces this risk. For example, women with an abnormal BRCA1 gene have an increased risk of developing ovarian cancer. However, if women with the abnormal gene are screened more often and have their ovaries removed when the risk of cancer seems elevated, their cause-specific hazard for ovarian cancer may be lower than in women without the abnormal gene.

Another example in which the marginal hazard and the cause-specific hazard differ is for AIDS as event in IDUs. In Figure 1.15 we saw that the Kaplan-Meier estimate was steeper for MSM than for IDUs. The Kaplan-Meier monotonically relates to the estimate of the cumulative hazard that censors individuals when they experience a competing event, which is the cause-specific hazard. Therefore, a similar difference is observed in the estimates of the AIDS-specific cumulative hazards in Figure 6.1. For the IDUs it is not an estimate of the marginal hazard, which we concluded by looking at the causes of death (see Table 1.2).

In both examples, the amount of informative censoring due to the competing risks differs by subgroup. If it is about the same in each group, relative cause-specific hazards are comparable to relative marginal hazards, even though cause-specific and marginal hazards differ in absolute value. This situation may be fairly common, but unfortunately it is an assumption that can not be verified based on the data.

If we have extra information, then we may be able to estimate the marginal distribution. In the IDU-MSM example, we may have information on CD4 T-cell count, which is the most important marker of AIDS progression. We can include such information as covariables in a model for the censoring time distribution and use censoring weights (see Section 1.5.1), or we can include it as covariables in a regression model. If the value of the information is categorical

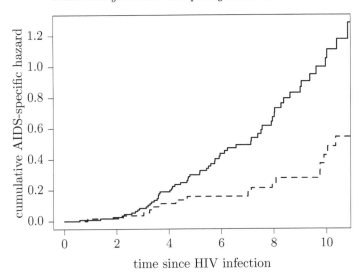

FIGURE 6.1
Cumulative AIDS-specific hazard for IDU (dashed line) and MSM (solid line).

and changes over time, another option is to include it via states in a multi-state model. Yet, whatever we do, there is no guarantee that it is sufficient to explain the censoring and make it non-informative.

We obtain a more detailed description of a disease process if we take intermediate events into account via a multi-state model. For example, if we want to quantify how the CCR5-Δ32 deletion changes progression to AIDS, and include the switch to SI as intermediate event, then we obtain more detailed information on the mechanism behind the protective effect of the deletion. Preferably, we define the states in such a way that the Markov assumption holds, which greatly simplifies analysis. Then, the transitions can be analysed as a nested sequence of competing risks settings. In each we quantify the transition-specific hazard—the multi-state equivalent of the cause-specific hazard—for all events that can occur next.

Prediction

For prediction we want to know the probability that an event happens within a certain time span. This probability is usually modeled as a function of covariables. In a competing risks setting, it not only depends on how the covariables relate to the event of interest, but also on how they relate to the competing event types. A change in covariable value can increase the cause-specific cumulative incidence not only by a direct etiologic mechanism, but also if it makes the other events less likely to occur. Hence, it may be better to speak of the impact of a covariable rather than of the effect. As a consequence, the cause-specific hazard for the event of interest does not suffice for the cumulative scale; we need to consider all cause-specific hazards. Compared to the effect on the cause-specific hazard, the direction of the impact on the cumulative scale may even be reversed (see Section 5.2.1).

An alternative is to use a regression model for the subdistribution hazard or directly for the cause-specific cumulative incidence. In these models, the impact on the cumulative scale of a change in covariable only depends on the parameter estimates for that specific event type. The advantage of such models is that, if we are only interested in the direction of the impact on the cumulative scale and not in the actual probabilities, we can restrict to reporting the parameter estimates.

The most common approach is to use a model that assumes proportionality on the subdistribution hazard, often called the Fine and Gray model [34]. Since the parameters incorporate the disturbing influence of the competing events on the cumulative probability, this model has sometimes been called a competing risks regression model (see e.g. the paper that is referred to in Exercise 6.2.5). The estimate of the subdistribution hazard incorporates the competing risks by ignoring them: individuals that experience a competing event are not censored but remain in the risk set. However, calling it a competing risks regression model may give the incorrect suggestion that the regression model for the cause-specific hazard ignores the competing risks issue and therefore does not apply in the presence of competing risks. Both models can be used in the competing risks setting, but the estimation method and the interpretation of the parameters differ.

A multi-state model is useful if we want to predict the flow of events. It can be used to predict the probability to be in some intermediate state, a probability that can go up and down over time. However, it is also useful to predict the cumulative probability to reach a final state based on time-updated information on the disease process, as reflected by intermediate states.

6.2 Exercises

1. On Page 183 we stated that the CCR5-Δ32 deletion decreases the marginal hazard of AIDS, which was defined as "the hazard of AIDS if other events do not prevent AIDS to occur". Why is it called a marginal hazard if a switch to SI phenotype can occur on the pathway from HIV infection to AIDS?

2. We want to compare time from HIV infection to AIDS between IDUs and MSM (Example 1 in Section 1.2.2). In our data set, many IDUs died before developing AIDS (see Section 1.6.2). In Figure 1.15 we plotted the Kaplan-Meier curve. If we combine both end points, AIDS and death, the curves in

Figure 6.2 are obtained. The difference between these curves is not significant based on the log-rank test (p-value 0.14). Under what assumptions can we interpret this as a comparison of the marginal distributions of time to AIDS between IDUs and MSM?

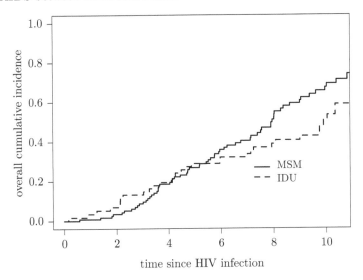

FIGURE 6.2
Estimate of cumulative incidence of combined end point death and AIDS.

3. Comment on the following statement

> When the ratio of the marginal hazards is the desired estimand and a regression model on the cause-specific hazard or subdistribution hazard is used, they can be considered ad hoc methods for estimating the ratio of the marginal hazards.

4. As explained on page 3, the definition of AIDS comprises a collection of diseases. After a first AIDS defining illness (the index diagnosis), individuals may develop other diseases that are also included in the AIDS definition.

   Kaposi's sarcoma (KS) is a tumor caused by the human herpesvirus type 8 (HHV8). In some individuals it is the index diagnosis, in others it occurs after another one and there are also individuals that die of AIDS without ever having had KS. Suppose that we ignore all other AIDS defining illnesses in our analyses and only consider KS as an event, also if another AIDS defining illness happened before. Can the hazard estimate thus obtained be interpreted as a marginal hazard of KS?

5. In a study on the effect of the use of β-blockers on prostate cancer

(PCa) [43], the authors used a proportional subdistribution hazards model for PCa-specific death, with other causes of death as competing event type. They found that individuals that used β-blockers had a lower subdistribution hazard for PCa-specific death. On the other hand, these individuals had an increased subdistribution hazard for other causes of death, such as cardiac mortality. In the discussion they address the question of whether this increased hazard for other CODs can explain the lower hazard for PCa-specific death. Comment on the following statement:

> To address this potential bias, we performed all analyses with the Fine and Gray competing risk regression model. In addition, we observed no increase in all-cause mortality among β-blocker users although other-cause mortality was higher, strengthening the interpretation of an association between the use of β-blockers and PCa-specific mortality.

6. The introduction of combination antiviral therapy (cART) has greatly changed the disease course from HIV infection to AIDS and death. In the search for the best moment to start cART, we investigated whether individuals who start cART in the first year after HIV infection ("early starters") have a different risk of treatment failure than individuals who start later, i.e. during chronic infection [113].

Treatment change and treatment interruption were treated as competing risks. In Figure 6.3, we plot the cause-specific cumulative incidence estimates for the three event types.

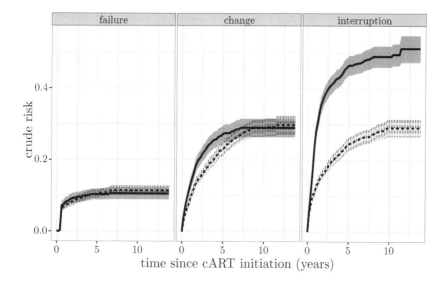

FIGURE 6.3

Cause-specific cumulative incidence (with 95% CI) by exposure group. Solid lines: early starters; dashed lines: late starters.

Contrary to expectation, we did not see a lower probability of treatment failure in the group of early starters. However, the early starters were much more likely to interrupt treatment. In order to investigate the influence of potential confounders, we fitted a proportional subdistribution hazards model that included risk group and age, amongst others. Results did not change much. The subdistribution hazard ratio for failure as end point for the early starters versus the late starters was 0.93 (95% CI 0.72-1.20). For treatment change and treatment interruption, the subdistribution hazard ratios were 1.06 (95% CI 0.91-1.24) and 1.54 (95% CI 1.33-1.79) respectively.

Comment on the following explanation for the lack of effect on treatment failure:

> It may be that individuals interrupt treatment because they are responding well to therapy, rather than simply because they are scheduled to do so. In that case, they would be less likely to fail treatment if they had not interrupted and the marginal hazard ratio of failing treatment in early versus chronic infection would be smaller than the one we report.

Bibliography

[1] Odd O. Aalen, Ørnulf Borgan, and Håkon K. Gjessing. *Survival and Event History Analysis*. Springer Verlag, New York, 2010.

[2] Odd O. Aalen and Søren Johansen. An empirical transition matrix for non-homogeneous Markov chains based on censored observations. *Scandinavian Journal of Statistics*, 5(3):141–150, 1978.

[3] Arthur Allignol, Martin Schumacher, and Jan Beyersmann. A note on variance estimation of the Aalen-Johansen estimator of the cumulative incidence function in competing risks, with a view towards left-truncated data. *Biometrical Journal*, 52(1):126–137, 2010.

[4] Arthur Allignol, Martin Schumacher, and Jan Beyersmann. Empirical transition matrix of multi-state models: The `etm` package. *Journal of Statistical Software*, 38(4):1–15, 2011. `http://www.jstatsoft.org/v38/i04`

[5] P. K. Andersen and N. Keiding. Interpretability and importance of functionals in competing risks and multistate models. *Statistics in Medicine*, 31(11-12):1074–1088, 2012.

[6] Per Kragh Andersen, Ørnulf Borgan, Richard D. Gill, and Niels Keiding. *Statistical Models Based on Counting Processes*. Springer Verlag, New York, 1993.

[7] Per Kragh Andersen and Niels Keiding. Multi-state models for event history analysis. *Statistical Methods in Medical Research*, 11(2):91–115, 2002.

[8] Ruta Bajorunaite and John P. Klein. Comparison of failure probabilities in the presence of competing risks. *Journal of Statistical Computation and Simulation*, 78(10):951–966, 2008.

[9] S. M. Bentzen, M. Vaeth, D. E. Pedersen, and J. Overgaard. Why actuarial estimates should be used in reporting late normal-tissue effects of cancer treatment ... now! *International Journal of Radiation Oncology * Biology * Physics*, 32(5):1531–1534, 1995.

[10] Rebecca A Betensky and David A Schoenfeld. Nonparametric estimation in a cure model with random cure times. *Biometrics*, 57(1):282–286, 2001.

[11] J. Beyersmann and M. Schumacher. Time-dependent covariates in the proportional subdistribution hazards model for competing risks. *Biostatistics*, 9(4):765–776, 2008.

[12] Jan Beyersmann, Arthur Allignol, and Martin Schumacher. *Competing Risks and Multistate Models with R*. Springer Verlag, New York, 2012.

[13] Jan Beyersmann and Martin Schumacher. Misspecified regression model for the subdistribution hazard of a competing risk. *Statistics in Medicine*, 26(7):1649–1651, 2007.

[14] K. Bhaskaran, B. Rachet, S. Evans, and L. Smeeth. Re: Helene Hartvedt Grytli, Morten Wang Fagerland, Sophie D. Fosså, Kristin Austlid Taskén. Association between use of β-blockers and prostate cancer-specific survival: a cohort study of 3561 prostate cancer patients with high-risk or metastatic disease. *European Urology*, 64(4):e86–87, 2013.

[15] Ø. Borgan and K. Liestøl. A note on confidence intervals and bands for the survival function based on transformations. *Scandinavian Journal of Statistics*, 17(1):35–41, 1990.

[16] Thomas M. Braun and Zheng Yuan. Comparing the small sample performance of several variance estimators under competing risks. *Statistics in Medicine*, 26(5):1170–1180, 2007.

[17] A. Bureau, S. Shiboski, and J. P. Hughes. Applications of continuous time hidden Markov models to the study of misclassified disease outcomes. *Statistics in Medicine*, 22(3):441–462, 2003.

[18] R. J. Caplan, T. F. Pajak, and J. D. Cox. Analysis of the probability and risk of cause-specific failure. *International Journal of Radiation Oncology * Biology * Physics*, 29(5):1183–1186, 1994.

[19] CASCADE Collaboration (Concerted Action on SeroConversion to AIDS and Death in Europe). Changes in the uptake of antiretroviral therapy and survival in people with known duration of HIV infection in Europe: results from CASCADE. *HIV Medicine*, 1(4):224–231, 2000.

[20] Wei-Hwa Chang and Weijing Wang. Regression analysis for cumulative incidence probability under competing risks. *Statistica Sinica*, 19(2):391–408, 2009.

[21] R. Chappell. Re: Caplan et al. IJROBP 29:1183-1186; 1994, and Bentzen et al. IJROBP 32:1531-1534; 1995. *International Journal of Radiation Oncology * Biology * Physics*, 36(4):988–989, 1996.

[22] R. Chappell. Competing risk analyses: how are they different and why should you care? *Clinical Cancer Research*, 18(8):2127–2129, 2012.

[23] G. Cortese and P. K. Andersen. Competing risks and time-dependent covariates. *Biometrical Journal*, 52(1):138–158, 2010.

[24] G. Cortese, T. A. Gerds, and P. K. Andersen. Comparing predictions among competing risks models with time-dependent covariates. *Statistics in Medicine*, 32(18):3089–3101, 2013.

[25] V. Coviello and M Boggess. Cumulative incidence estimation in the presence of competing risks. *Stata Journal*, 4(2):103–112, 2004.

[26] Somnath Datta and Glen A. Satten. Validity of the Aalen-Johansen estimators of stage occupation probabilities and Nelson-Aalen estimators of integrated transition hazards for non-Markov models. *Statistics & Probability Letters*, 55(4):403–411, 2001.

[27] Somnath Datta and Glen A. Satten. Estimation of integrated transition hazards and stage occupation probabilities for non-Markov systems under dependent censoring. *Biometrics*, 58(4):792–802, 2002.

[28] Liesbeth C. de Wreede, Marta Fiocco, and Hein Putter. mstate: An R package for the analysis of competing risks and multi-state models. *Journal of Statistical Software*, 38(7):1–30, 2011. http://www.jstatsoft.org/v38/i07

[29] E. Deslandes and S. Chevret. Joint modeling of multivariate longitudinal data and the dropout process in a competing risk setting: application to ICU data. *BMC Medical Research Methodology*, 10:69, 2010. http://www.biomedcentral.com/1471-2288/10/69

[30] Bradley Efron. The two sample problem with censored data. In Lucien M. Le Cam and Jerzy Neyman, editors, *Proceedings of the Fifth Berkeley Symposium On Mathematical Statistics and Probability*, pages 831–853, New-York, 1967. Prentice-Hall.

[31] Nicole Ferguson, Somnath Datta, and Guy Brock. msSurv: An R package for nonparametric estimation of multistate models. *Journal of Statistical Software*, 50(14):1–24, 2012. http://www.jstatsoft.org/v50/i14

[32] J. P. Fine, H. Jiang, and R. Chappell. On semi-competing risks data. *Biometrika*, 88(4):907–919, 2001.

[33] Jason P. Fine. Analysing competing risks data with transformation models. *Journal of the Royal Statistical Society. Series B, Statistical methodology*, 61(4):817–830, 1999.

[34] Jason P. Fine and Robert J. Gray. A proportional hazards model for the subdistribution of a competing risk. *Journal of the American Statistical Association*, 94(446):496–509, 1999.

[35] Jeffrey J Gaynor, Eric J Feuer, Claire C Tan, Danny H Wu, Claudia R Little, David J Straus, Bayard D Clarkson, and Murray F Brennan. On the use of cause-specific failure and conditional failure probabilities: examples from clinical oncology data. *Journal of the American Statistical Association*, 88(422):400–409, 1993.

[36] Thomas A. Gerds, Thomas H. Scheike, and Per K. Andersen. Absolute risk regression for competing risks: interpretation, link functions, and prediction. *Statistics in Medicine*, 31(29):3921–3930, 2012.

[37] Ronald B. Geskus. Cause-specific cumulative incidence estimation and the fine and gray model under both left truncation and right censoring. *Biometrics*, 67(1):39–49, 2011.

[38] Ronald B. Geskus, Frank A. Miedema, Jaap Goudsmit, Peter Reiss, Hanneke Schuitemaker, and Roel A. Coutinho. Prediction of residual time to AIDS and death based on markers and cofactors. *Journal of Acquired Immune Deficiency Syndromes and Human Retrovirology*, 32(5):514–521, 2003.

[39] T. A. Gooley, W. Leisenring, J. Crowley, and B.E. Storer. Estimation of failure probabilities in the presence of competing risks: New representations of old estimators. *Statistics in Medicine*, 18(6):695–706, 1999.

[40] Robert J. Gray. A class of k-sample tests for comparing the cumulative incidence of a competing risk. *Annals of Statistics*, 16(3):1141–1154, 1988.

[41] Sander Greenland, James M. Robins, and Judea Pearl. Confounding and collapsity in causal inference. *Statistical Science*, 14(1):29–46, 1999.

[42] P. Groeneboom, M. H. Maathuis, and J. A. Wellner. Current status data with competing risks: limiting distribution of the MLE. *Annals of Statistics*, 36(3):1064–1089, 2008.

[43] H. H. Grytli, M. W. Fagerland, S. D. Fosså, and K. A. Taskén. Association between use of β-blockers and prostate cancer-specific survival: a cohort study of 3561 prostate cancer patients with high-risk or metastatic disease. *European Urology*, 65(6):635–641, 2014.

[44] R. G. Gutierrez. In the spotlight: Competing-risks regression. *The Stata News*, 25(4):1–2, 2010.

[45] Frank E. Harrell Jr. *Regression Modeling Strategies*. Springer Verlag, New York, 2001.

[46] S. R. Hinchliffe and P. C. Lambert. Flexible parametric modelling of cause-specific hazards to estimate cumulative incidence functions. *BMC Medical Research Methodology*, 13:13, 2013. http://www.biomedcentral.com/1471-2288/13/13

[47] D. R. Hoover, A. Muñoz, V. Carey, J. M. G. Taylor, M. Vanraden, J. S. Chmiel, and L. Kingsley. Using events from dropouts in nonparametric survival function estimation with application to incubation of AIDS. *Journal of the American Statistical Association*, 421(1):37–43, 1993.

[48] Chanelle J. Howe, Stephen R. Cole, Joan S. Chmiel, and Alvaro Muñoz. Limitation of inverse probability-of-censoring weights in estimating survival in the presence of strong selection bias. *American Journal of Epidemiology*, 173(5):569–577, 2011.

[49] F. B. Hu, J. Goldberg, D. Hedeker, B. R. Flay, and M. A. Pentz. Comparison of population-averaged and subject-specific approaches for analyzing repeated binary outcomes. *American Journal of Epidemiology*, 147(7):694–703, 1998.

[50] S. Iacobelli and B. Carstensen. Multiple time scales in multi-state models. *Statistics in Medicine*, 32(30):5315–5327, 2013.

[51] J. D. Kalbfleisch and R. L. Prentice. *The Statistical Analysis of Failure Time Data, Second Edition*. Wiley, New York, 2002.

[52] Niels Keiding and Richard D. Gill. Random truncation models and Markov prcesses. *Annals of Statistics*, 18(2):582–602, 1990.

[53] Haesook T Kim. Cumulative incidence in competing risks data and competing risks regression analysis. *Clinical Cancer Research*, 13(2):559–565, 2007.

[54] J. P. Klein. Small sample moments of some estimators of the variance of the Kaplan-Meier and Nelson-Aalen estimators. *Scandinavian Journal of Statistics*, 18(4):333–340, 1991.

[55] J. P. Klein and M. L. Moeschberger. *Survival Analysis, Techniques for Censored and Truncated Data*. Springer Verlag, New York, 1997.

[56] John P. Klein. Modeling competing risks in cancer studies. *Statistics in Medicine*, 25(6):1015–1034, 2006.

[57] John P. Klein and Per Kragh Andersen. Regression modeling of competing risks data based on pseudovalues of the cumulative incidence function. *Biometrics*, 61(1):223–229, 2005.

[58] John P. Klein and Ruta Bajorunaite. Inference for competing risks. In N. Balakrishnan and C. R. Rao, editors, *Handbook of Statistics*, volume 23, pages 291–311. Elsevier Science, Amsterdam, 2004.

[59] John P. Klein, Niels Keiding, and Edward A. Copelan. Plotting summary predictions in multistate survival models: probabilities of relapse and death in remission for bone marrow transplanation patients. *Statistics in Medicine*, 13(22):2315–2332, 1994.

[60] Maria Kohl, Max Plischke, Karen Leffondrè, and Georg Heinze. PSHREG: A SAS macro for proportional and nonproportional hazards regression. *Computer Methods and Programs in Biomedicine*, 118(2):218–233, 2015.

[61] M. T. Koller, H. Raatz, E. W. Steyerberg, and M. Wolbers. Competing risks and the clinical community: irrelevance or ignorance? *Statistics in Medicine*, 31(11-12):1089–1097, 2012.

[62] David Kraus. Adaptive Neyman's smooth tests of homogeneity of two samples of survival data. *Journal of Statistical Planning and Inference*, 139(10):3559–3569, 2009.

[63] M. G. Larson and G. E. Dinse. A mixture model for the regression analysis of competing risks data. *Journal of the Royal Statistical Society. Series C, Applied Statistics*, 34(3):201–211, 1985.

[64] A. Latouche, J. Beyersmann, and J. P. Fine. Comments on 'analysing and interpreting competing risk data'. *Statistics in Medicine*, 26(19):3676–9; author reply 3679–80, 2007.

[65] Chenxi Li, Robert J. Gray, and Jason P. Fine. Reader reaction: On variance estimation for the fine-gray model. Technical Report 29, The University of North Carolina at Chapel Hill, Department of Biostatistics, 2012. http://biostats.bepress.com/uncbiostat/art29

[66] J. Li, J. Le-Rademacher, and M. J. Zhang. Weighted comparison of two cumulative incidence functions with R-CIFsmry package. *Computer Methods and Programs in Biomedicine*, 116(3):205–214, 2014.

[67] Kung-Yee Liang and Scott L. Zeger. Longitudinal data analysis using generalized linear models. *Biometrika*, 73(1):13–22, 1986.

[68] D. Y. Lin. Non-parametric inference for cumulative incidence functions in competing risks studies. *Statistics in Medicine*, 16(8):901–910, 1997.

[69] Mary Lunn and Don McNeil. Applying Cox regression to competing risks. *Biometrics*, 51(2):524–532, 1995.

[70] Y. Matsuyama and T. Yamaguchi. Estimation of the marginal survival time in the presence of dependent competing risks using inverse probability of censoring weighted (IPCW) methods. *Pharmaceutical Statistics*, 7(3):202–214, 2008.

[71] L. Meira-Machado. Inference for non-Markov multi-state models: an overview. *REVSTAT Statistical Journal*, 9(1):83–98, 2011.

[72] L. Meira-Machado, J. de Una-Alvarez, and C. Cadarso-Suarez. Non-parametric estimation of transition probabilities in a non-Markov illness-death model. *Lifetime Data Analysis*, 12(3):325–344, 2006.

[73] Johannes Mertsching. A comparison of different approaches to nonparametric inference for subdistributions. Master's thesis in mathematics, University of Amsterdam, 2013. `https://esc.fnwi.uva.nl/thesis/`

[74] M. Nicolaie, H. V. Houwelingen, and H. Putter. Vertical modeling: Analysis of competing risks data with missing causes of failure. *Statistical Methods in Medical Research*, Epub ahead of print; doi: 10.1177/0962280211432067, 2011.

[75] Megan Othus, Bart Barlogie, Michael L. LeBlanc, and John J. Crowley. Cure models as a useful statistical tool for analyzing survival. *Clinical Cancer Research*, 18(14):3731–3736, 2012.

[76] Yingwei Peng and Keith B. G. Dear. A nonparametric mixture model for cure rate estimation. *Biometrics*, 56(1):237–243, 2000.

[77] Melania Pintilie. Analysing and interpreting competing risk data. *Statistics in Medicine*, 26(6):1360–1367, 2007.

[78] Núria Porta-Bleda. *Interval-censored semi-competing risks data: a novel approach for modelling bladder cancer.* Ph.D. dissertation, Universitat Politècnica de Catalunya, 2010. `http://hdl.handle.net/10803/6532`

[79] R. L. Prentice, J. D. Kalbfleisch, A. V. Peterson, N. Flournoy, V. T. Farewell, and N. E. Breslow. The analysis of failure times in the presence of competing risks. *Biometrics*, 34(4):541–554, 1978.

[80] Maria Prins and Paul J. Veugelers for the European Seroconverter Study and the Tricontinental Seroconverter Study. Comparison of progression and non-progression in injecting drug users and homosexual men with documented dates of HIV-1 seroconversion. *AIDS*, 11(5):621–631, 1997.

[81] H. Putter, M. Fiocco, and R. B. Geskus. Tutorial in biostatistics: competing risks and multi-state models. *Statistics in Medicine*, 26(11):2389–2430, 2007.

[82] H. Putter and H. C. van Houwelingen. Frailties in multi-state models: Are they identifiable? Do we need them? *Statistical Methods in Medical Research*, Epub ahead of print; doi: 10.1177/0962280211424665, 2011.

[83] R Core Team. *R: A Language and Environment for Statistical Computing.* R Foundation for Statistical Computing, Vienna, Austria, 2015. `http://www.r-project.org`

[84] Dimitris Rizopoulos. *Joint Models for Longitudinal and Time-to-Event Data.* Chapman and Hall/CRC, Boca Raton, 2012.

[85] J. M. Robins and D. M. Finkelstein. Correcting for noncompliance and dependent censoring in an AIDS Clinical Trial with inverse probability of censoring weighted (IPCW) log-rank tests. *Biometrics*, 56(3):779–788, 2000.

[86] P. K. Ruan and R. J. Gray. Analyses of cumulative incidence functions via non-parametric multiple imputation. *Statistics in Medicine*, 27(27):5709–5724, 2008.

[87] J. M. Satagopan, L. Ben-Porat, M. Berwick, M. Robson, D. Kutler, and A. D. Auerbach. A note on competing risks in survival data analysis. *British Journal of Cancer*, 91(7):1229–1235, 2004.

[88] Glen A. Satten and Somnath Datta. The Kaplan-Meier estimator as an inverse-probability-of-censoring weighted average. *American Statistician*, 55(3):207–210, 2001.

[89] Glen A. Satten, Somnath Datta, and James Robins. Estimating the marginal survival function in the presence of time dependent covariates. *Statistics & Probability Letters*, 54(4):397–403, 2001.

[90] Glen A. Satten and Ira M. Longini. Markov chains with measurement error: Estimating the "true" course of a marker of the progression of human immunodeficiency virus disease. *Journal of the Royal Statistical Society. Series C, Applied Statistics*, 45(3):275–309, 1996.

[91] Thomas H. Scheike and Mei-Jie Zhang. Direct modelling of regression effects for transition probabilities in multistate models. *Scandinavian Journal of Statistics*, 34(1):17–32, 2007.

[92] Thomas H. Scheike, Mei-Jie Zhang, and Thomas A. Gerds. Predicting cumulative incidence probability by direct binomial regression. *Biometrika*, 95(1):205–220, 2008.

[93] Pao-sheng Shen. The product-limit estimate as an inverse-probability-weighted average. *Communications in Statistics*, 32(6):1119–1133, 2003.

[94] Pao-sheng Shen. Proportional subdistribution hazards regression for left-truncated competing risks data. *Journal of Nonparametric Statistics*, 23(4):885–895, 2011.

[95] Meredith S. Shiels, Stephen R. Cole, Joan S. Chmiel, Joseph Margolick, Jeremy Martinson, Zuo-Feng Zhang, and Lisa P. Jacobson. A comparison of ad hoc methods to account for non-cancer AIDS and deaths as competing risks when estimating the effect of HAART on incident cancer AIDS among HIV-infected men. *Journal of Clinical Epidemiology*, 63(4):459–467, 2010.

[96] C. Spitoni, M. Verduijn, and H. Putter. Estimation and asymptotic theory for transition probabilities in Markov renewal multi-state models. *International Journal of Biostatistics*, 8(1):23, 2012.

[97] Ewout W. Steyerberg. *Clinical Prediction Models*. Springer Verlag, New York, 2009.

[98] Judy P. Sy and Jeremy M. G. Taylor. Estimation in a Cox proportional hazards cure model. *Biometrics*, 56(1):227–236, 2000.

[99] B. C. Tai, I. R. White, V. Gebski, and D. Machin. On the issue of "multiple" first failures in competing risks analysis. *Statistics in Medicine*, 21(15):2243–2255, 2002.

[100] Terry M. Therneau and Patricia M. Grambsch. *Modeling survival data: extending the Cox model*. Springer Verlag, New York, 2000.

[101] H. Thijs, G. Molenberghs, B. Michiels, G. Verbeke, and D. Curran. Strategies to fit pattern-mixture models. *Biostatistics*, 3(2):245–265, Jun 2002.

[102] Wei-Yann Tsai. Testing the assumption of independence of truncation time and failure time. *Biometrika*, 77(1):169–177, 1990.

[103] A. A. Tsiatis. A nonidentifiability aspect of the problem of competing risks. *Proceedings of the National Academy of Sciences of the United States of America*, 72(1):20–22, 1975.

[104] J. van der Helm, R. Geskus, C. Sabin, L Meyer, J del Amo, G. Chêne, M. Dorrucci, R Muga, K. Porter, and M. Prins on behalf of CASCADE Collaboration in EuroCoord. Effect of HCV infection on cause-specific mortality after HIV seroconversion, before and after 1997. *Gastroenterology*, 144(4):751–760, 2013.

[105] Mark J. van der Laan and James M. Robins. *Unified Methods for Censored Longitudinal Data and Causality*. Springer Verlag, New York, 2003.

[106] Helena J. van der Pal, Elvira C. van Dalen, Evelien van Delden, Irma W. van Dijk, Wouter E. Kok, Ronald B. Geskus, Elske Sieswerda, Foppe Oldenburger, Caro C. Koning, Flora E. van Leeuwen, Huib N. Caron, and Leontien C. Kremer. High risk of symptomatic cardiac events in childhood cancer survivors. *Journal of Clinical Oncology*, 30(13):1429–1437, 2012.

[107] N. van Geloven, R. B. Geskus, B. W. Mol, and A. H. Zwinderman. Correcting for the dependent competing risk of treatment using inverse probability of censoring weighting and copulas in the estimation of natural conception chances. *Statistics in Medicine*, 33(26):4671–4680, 2014.

[108] H. C. van Houwelingen and H. Putter. *Dynamic Prediction in Clinical Survival Analysis*. Chapman and Hall/CRC Press, Boca Raton, 2011.

[109] M. Wolbers, P. Blanche, M. T. Koller, J. C. Witteman, and T. A. Gerds. Concordance for prognostic models with competing risks. *Biostatistics*, 15(3):526–539, 2014.

[110] M. Wolbers, M. T. Koller, J. C. Witteman, and E. W. Steyerberg. Prognostic models with competing risks: methods and application to coronary risk prediction. *Epidemiology*, 20(4):555–561, 2009.

[111] Xu Zhang, Mei-Jie Zhang, and Jason P. Fine. A mass redistribution algorithm for right-censored and left-truncated time to event data. *Journal of Statistical Planning and Inference*, 139(9):3329–3339, 2009.

[112] B. Zhou, J. Fine, and G. Laird. Goodness-of-fit test for proportional subdistribution hazards model. *Statistics in Medicine*, 32(22):3804–3811, 2013.

[113] D. Zugna, R. B. Geskus, B. De Stavola, M. Rosinska, B. Bartmeyer, F. Boufassa, M. L. Chaix, A. Babiker, K. Porter, and the CASCADE Collaboration in EUROCOORD. Time to virological failure, treatment change and interruption for individuals treated within 12 months of HIV seroconversion and in chronic infection. *Antiviral Therapy*, 17(6):1039–1048, 2012.

Appendix: Answers to Exercises

Chapter 1: Basic Concepts

1. The left panel shows the probability (solid line) and the hazard (dashed line). The probability curve shows that the most likely age of death is around 80 years. The hazard increases rapidly after 60 years: the older you are, the more likely you are to die within the coming year. The right panel shows the survival curve. The slope of the survival curve corresponds to the probability: the steeper the curve, the more individuals die at that age.

2. Censoring is not necessarily informative when it is caused by an intervening, competing, event. However, it is informative if ovarian cancer and breast cancer are partly the consequence of the same biological process. This example was inspired by a statement in Satagopan *et al.* [87, p.1230].

3. The Kaplan-Meier is a valid estimator of the marginal distribution if all censoring is non-informative. Removing individuals from the risk set before they experience the competing event removes the competing risk, but does not solve the problem of informative censoring.

4. Strategy A may seem to be an attractive one. It includes all observed events. However, only individuals that developed AIDS after they left the PHS are given extra follow-up, not the ones for whom AIDS was not observed after their last visit at the PHS. Since individuals with and without later events are not treated equally, the strategy gives a biased estimate.

   Strategy B treats all information on individuals that left the PHS in the same way. It is a valid strategy if we can assume that all individuals that left the study and for whom we did not observe a subsequent AIDS diagnosis were still AIDS-free at 1-1-1997; hence it assumes that the acquired information from the hospitals and the AIDS registry is complete[1].

   Strategy C is biased. Several individuals developed AIDS shortly after their last visit. If we remove individuals from the risk set just before they develop AIDS, the estimate of the survival curve will be too high. Note that, when saying that censoring is informative, we use extra information

---

[1] We ignore that two individuals died after they had left the PHS for reasons that were not related to AIDS.

after the censoring time; we are not able to see this based on the time-to-censoring data alone. Several individuals developed AIDS shortly after they had left the PHS because these individuals were not really lost to follow-up. They continued to be seen in one of the hospitals in Amsterdam. Data from these hospitals has been linked to the ACS data.

D is similar to B. The only difference is that we use 1-1-1993 as date of analysis. If the AIDS registry is complete, it should give unbiased results, similar to strategy B. Of course, if we have follow-up until 1997, we would throw away information by restricting our analysis to data until 1993. Hence, strategy B is more efficient.

Strategy E was used as the general strategy in a multi-center study that included data from the ACS [80]. It was hoped to prevent the bias that arose by excluding AIDS diagnoses that occurred in the hospital just after individuals had left the study. At the same time, completeness with respect to AIDS diagnosis for the individuals that had left the study is only assumed during the first two years.

In Figure A.1, the Kaplan-Meier plots are compared.

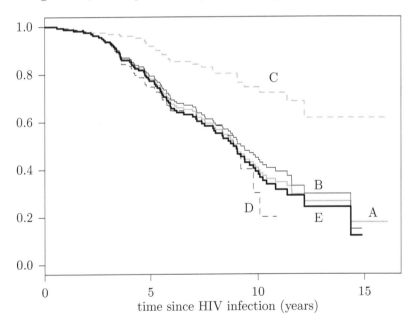

FIGURE A.1
Kaplan-Meier plots. A: grey solid line; B: black solid thin line; C: grey dashed line; D: black dashed line; E:black solid thick line.

1) A and B: the Kaplan-Meier from B is always higher than the one from A. In B, individuals that were censored before 1997 and did not develop

AIDS are given extra follow-up time until 1997. Hence, at any time the number at risk is larger[2]. If the number at risk $r(t)$ is larger, $1/r(t)$ is smaller and $(1 - 1/r(t))$ is larger. Since the Kaplan-Meier is a product of such terms, the estimated survival curve moves upward.

2) A and C: In strategy C, we have fewer events, but also less follow-up time. These effects work in opposite direction in the Kaplan-Meier and we cannot say in general how the Kaplan-Meiers compare. However, in this specific data set many events happened just after having stopped follow-up at the ACS. If we don't include the extra information, the Kaplan-Meier is considerably higher.

3) B and D: If the AIDS registry is complete, no systematic difference is expected. Jumps are somewhat larger in D because we use less information.

4) B and E: If both strategies are valid, we do not expect any systematic difference. However, we cannot say which one is higher for a specific data set, because both events and follow-up time differ between the methods.

A clear overview of different strategies and their possible biases is given in [47].

5. The censoring is informative for time to AIDS if we do not correct for age or calendar period. Individuals that were censored shortly after HIV infection are the ones that became HIV infected after 1990. They were on average older. Since time to AIDS is shorter for older individuals, those who were censored early after HIV infection have on average a shorter time to AIDS than the individuals that remained in follow-up for a longer period.

6. The statement is not correct. We cannot tell from the data on events and censorings (i.e. dropouts) whether censoring is non-informative. A high dropout rate may be explained by study design or characteristics of the population from which the women were sampled. It does not tell whether women with a lower probability of conception are more likely to drop out of that study.

   The lack of observed trend can also correspond with the situation in which women with a low probability of conception are more likely to drop out in studies with a high dropout rate. This would give an upward bias in the observed pregnancy rate. If at the same time the probability of conception is lower on average in these studies, the observed data may show a constant pregnancy rate.

   If the bias due to informative dropout and the true pregnancy rate were the same in all studies, we would also observe a constant pregnancy rate, but this estimate would be biased.

7. We want to estimate and compare the marginal distribution of side effects.

---

[2]It may be equal in the very beginning of the time scale, until the first censoring due to loss to follow-up.

The comparison is fair if we can assume that side effects are equally likely to occur in individuals who stay in the hospital as in individuals that have been discharged, i.e. if discharge is non-informative with respect to the occurrence of side effects.

8. Since the data that was used is different—situation (II) was excluded in study A—survival curve estimates will differ as well. Study A gives biased results. The reason is that the criterion that determines whether an individual could enter the study (being AIDS free) is not independent of the end point (death). Since they had to be AIDS free when they entered the study, they could not be too close to death. Compared to individuals with the same time since HIV infection that had been in follow-up from HIV infection onwards, their hazard of death was smaller.

9* We apply the delta method to var$\{\log \widehat{F}(t)\}$ to obtain

$$\text{var}\{\log \widehat{F}(t)\} = \frac{\text{var}\{\widehat{F}(t)\}}{\{\widehat{F}(t)\}^2} \, .$$

The expression on the log scale now follows from $\widehat{F}(t) = \exp\{\log \widehat{F}(t)\}$.

For the expression on the log-log scale, we apply the delta method to var$[\log\{-\log \widehat{F}(t)\}]$. Note that the derivative of $f(x) = \log\{-\log(x)\}$ is $1/\{\log(x) \times x\}$. Next we use $\widehat{F}(t) = \exp(-\exp[\log\{-\log \widehat{F}(t)\}])$.

Chapter 2: Competing Risks; Nonparametric Estimation

1. Yes, this holds generally. Both estimators have the same numerator, whereas $r^*(t) \geq r(t)$. Therefore, the estimator of the cause-specific hazard is always larger than the estimator of the subdistribution hazard[3], and the same holds for the cumulative sum.

2. The cause-specific hazard is commonly defined as the hazard in the *presence* of competing risks. The hazard in the absence of competing risks is usually called the marginal hazard, net hazard or simply the hazard.

The statement has been copied from [77, p.1362]. Latouche *et al.*[64] replied:

> Pintilie's work has the potential to further obscure the issues ...Our main critique concerns the inaccurate assertion: "When modelling the cause specific hazard, one performs the analysis under the assumption that the competing risks do not exist".

---

[3] They are equal until the first competing event occurs.

3. No, the overall hazard is equal to a weighted sum of subdistribution hazards according to

$$\sum_{e=1}^{K} \lambda_e(t) = \sum_{e=1}^{K} \frac{\overline{F_e}(t)}{\overline{F}(t)} h_e(t).$$

This immediately follows from relation (2.12) on Page 63.

The denominator in the subdistribution hazard is always equal to or larger than the denominator in the cause-specific hazard: only individuals that experience the event of interest leave the risk set, whereas in the cause-specific hazard individuals leave the risk set with any event type. In order to come up with the same sum, we need to multiply by terms $\frac{\overline{F_e}(t)}{\overline{F}(t)} \geq 0$.

Note that the sum of the subdistribution probabilities is equal to the overall probability (see (2.6)).

4. In competing risks settings, we do not want to compare Kaplan-Meier cumulative incidence curves. However, the standard log-rank test is a valid test to test for equality of cause-specific hazards. The statement is adapted from Kim [53, p.562].

5. The Kaplan-Meier is obtained as

$$\widehat{\overline{F}}(t) = \prod_{t_{(j)} \leq t} \left\{ 1 - \frac{d_{\text{AIDS}}(t_{(j)})}{r(t_{(j)})} \right\}$$

This expression completely determines the estimate of the AIDS-specific hazard $\widehat{\lambda}_{\text{AIDS}}(t_{(i)}) = d_{\text{AIDS}}(t_{(i)})/r(t_{(i)})$ via relation (1.3). Therefore, the Kaplan-Meier allows us to conclude that the AIDS-specific hazard is different for IDU and MSM. However, if we want to conclude upon the difference in cause-specific hazards, it is better to plot and compare the cumulative AIDS-specific hazards for both groups (see Figure 6.1). This prevents misinterpretation as a marginal quantity.

6. On Page 33 it is shown that the overall Kaplan-Meier $\widehat{\overline{F}}^{\text{PL}}(t_{(i)}-)$ is equal to $r(t_{(i)})/N$. Combining this with (2.15), we see that the jump size in the Aalen-Johansen estimator is equal to $d_k(t_{(i)})/N$, which is equal to the jump size in the ECDF form.

7. $\widehat{A_1}$ is an estimate of the overall cumulative incidence. It is equal to one minus the Kaplan-Meier for overall survival.
$\widehat{A_2}$ estimates the marginal distribution of time to the cause of interest, but only if the competing risks occur as a consequence of independent mechanisms.
$\widehat{A_3}$ is an estimate of the cause-specific cumulative incidence.

8. The observation that both curves are almost the same is correct. However, this is not a general property, not even when censoring due to the

competing event is non-informative. The Kaplan-Meier and the estimator of the CE-specific cumulative incidence quantify different aspects. See the example with discharge and staphylococcus infection as competing risks, in which non-informative censoring due to discharge may be a reasonable assumption.

The reason that both curves are very similar is because there is little mortality due to other causes, at least during the first 20 years, when most of the symptomatic cardiac events occur. Also note that on one hand it is said that death due to other causes may not be related to CE events, whereas on the other hand it is called "informative censoring". The statement was inspired by a similar one on breast cancer and ovarian cancer in Satagopan *et al.* [87, p.1234].

9. The comparison does not tell us anything on the reason for the gender difference in relapse-specific cumulative incidence. The Kaplan-Meier is supposed to estimate the marginal distribution, which quantifies a different aspect than the cause-specific cumulative incidence. See the example with discharge and staphylococcus infection as competing risks. Moreover, the Kaplan-Meier is a valid estimator only if DOC is noninformative for relapse. If DOC were informative for relapse, it does not quantify what would happen if DOC did not exist. The time-to-event data does not provide the information to determine the relation between DOC and relapse. For example, an extreme scenario which cannot be excluded based on the data is that every person that died would have progressed on the next day. This would be the same as combining the two event types and adding the cause-specific cumulative incidences of relapse and death. Then, the estimated marginal cumulative incidence curve for the males will become almost similar to the one for the females.

The reason that the Kaplan-Meier and the estimate of the cause-specific incidence are almost the same is because there is little mortality due to other causes, at least during the first 40 months, when most of the relapses occur.

The Kaplan-Meier does give information on the cause-specific hazards (see Exercise 2.8.5). We can conclude that females have a higher relapse-specific hazard than males and females have a lower DOC-specific hazard than males.

This exercise was inspired by the PhD thesis of Porta-Bleda [78, p.32]. In the thesis it is shown that the difference by gender is not explained by smoking status.

Chapter 3: Intermediate Events; Nonparametric Estimation

1. The expression in (3.6) is the Aalen-Johansen estimator for the competing risks setting. It assumes that individuals cannot leave the state as defined

by the event. If individuals can leave the state, an extra term needs to be included, as in (3.7).

2. We need to split the state "AIDS/SI" into two. One can be reached from "SI", the other from "AIDS". The resulting directed graph in shown in Figure A.2.

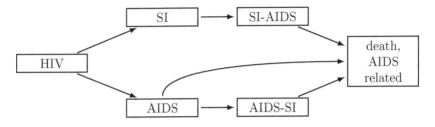

FIGURE A.2
Multi-state model; SI, AIDS and death are possible states and the sequence in which SI and AIDS occur can influence mortality.

3. It does not make any difference for the Nelson-Aalen estimator of the cumulative transition hazard. However, the estimator of the transition probability changes if censoring due to mortality is treated as a competing event. The situation is similar to the competing risks setting: the estimator of the cause-specific hazard is not affected by the assumption with respect to censoring, but the estimators of net risk and crude risk are not the same.

4. There are three single states that are not initial, SI, AIDS and death. The maximum number of transitions an individual can have is three as well. Individuals that have fewer than three events have empty values in some of the columns. The data format is shown in Table A.1. We use the notation NA for empty cells. Since everyone starts in the state "HIV", there is no need to specify a column for X^0.

TABLE A.1
Time and status information from four example individuals in the `aidssi2` data set, in time-ordered wide format

patnr	t^0	t^1	X^1	t^2	X^2	t^3	X^3	C
14	0.00	NA	NA	NA	NA	NA	NA	5.05
3	1.81	2.23	AIDS	2.26	death	NA	NA	NA
15	1.80	10.20	AIDS	NA	NA	NA	NA	12.93
8	2.80	8.61	SI	11.46	AIDS	11.94	death	NA
⋮	⋮	⋮	⋮	⋮	⋮	⋮	⋮	

5. All the transitions that leave from the HIV state are state occupation probabilities, i.e. transitions 1 and 2.

6. Figure 3.6 plots the estimate of the probability to be alive with AIDS over time, given that one is AIDS free at four years after HIV infection, but with a virus that has switched to SI phenotype. Figure 3.5 plots the estimate for those that were in state SI at time 0. Nobody was in state SI at time zero, but as we explained on Page 114, this is not a problem for the estimate of the transition probability. It is the interpretation that becomes less straightforward. It can be interpreted as the probability at the first moment that individuals can enter the SI state (which can be arbitrarily close to zero if the distributions are continuous). Since the curve returns to zero, it can also be interpreted as the probability from the next moment when individuals are observed to enter the SI state. But whatever s in $\widehat{P}_{23}(s,t)$ refers to, it is smaller than four years and hence the estimate is different.

7. We can obtain this estimate by only considering the first outgoing transitions from the AIDS state. In practice, this can be realized by making AIDS/SI an absorbing state, which creates a competing risks setting.

8. We show it for the simpler illness-death model, but the same argument holds for the curves in Figure 3.9. In the illness-death model, state 2 is absorbing. We estimate $P_{02}(s,t)$ via the Kaplan-Meier and the Aalen-Johansen estimator. The Kaplan-Meier jumps at each observed death time. For the Aalen-Johansen estimator we look at (3.8). Each of the two components is a sum of terms, the first over $u < t$, the second over $u \leq t$. For the second component, it changes value over t when a new term is added. This happens when $\widehat{\lambda}_{02}(t)$ is larger than zero, i.e. when there is an observed transition from 0 to 2. The first component changes value if $\widehat{P}_{12}(u+,t)$ changes value. From (3.6) we see that a change in $\widehat{P}_{12}(u+,t)$ is determined by $\widehat{\lambda}_{12}(t)$. Hence, jumps are determined by transitions from each of the two non-absorbing states to death, i.e. the observed death times.

9. In principle it is possible that the curves cross. Each curve refers to a different group of individuals: those that are in state SI at 2, 3 etc. years after HIV infection. It may be that individuals that enter the SI state between 2 and 3 years and are still in state SI at three years have a much faster progression to death than the individuals that were in the SI state at two years. Such phenomenon would indicate a violation of the Markov assumption, because the transition rate depends on the time of entry into that state.

Chapter 4: Regression; Cause-Specific/Transition Hazard

1. Statement I: With the commonly used definition, a cause-specific model quantifies the effect of a covariable on an event *in the presence of* competing risks. The statement is correct insofar as the comparison between the combined end point and a specific event in the presence of competing risks is concerned.

   Statement II: A cause-specific Cox regression indeed treats competing events as censored. But competing risks are not ignored with respect to the interpretation of the estimates.

   The statement resembles the one in Exercise 2 from Chapter 2. Of course, one can use another definition of cause-specific hazard, making it correspond with marginal hazard, but that is not recommended because it will generate confusion.

   The statements were adapted from Kim [53, p.559 and p.565].

2. (a) In principle we can choose any value in the cell with the three dots, but the interpretation of the parameters depends on the choice that is made. We use the value 20.

   (b) The following model is fitted

   $$\log\left\{\frac{P(Y = \text{yes}|X)}{1 - P(Y = \text{yes}|X)}\right\} = b_0 + b_1 X_1 + b_2 X_2 + b_3 X_3$$

   (c) In Table A.2 we give the effects on the logit scale for the three example individuals. We assume the reference value for the BRCA1 gene. i)

   TABLE A.2
   Effects on logit scale for three
   women

effect on logit scale	
No:	$b_0 + b_2 \times 20$
Yes, age 20:	$b_0 + b_1 + b_2 \times 20$
Yes, age 35:	$b_0 + b_1 + b_2 \times 35$

   The odds ratio of breast cancer for women who became pregnant at the age of 20 versus non-pregnant women is $\exp(b_1)$. ii) b_2 quantifies the effect of age at pregnancy. The odds ratio for the third woman compared to the second (age 35 versus age 20) is $\exp(b_2 \times 15)$. iii) The odds ratio for the third woman compared to the first is $\exp(b_1 + b_2 \times 15)$.

   In principle we can choose any age value at the dots, as long as it is the same for all women that did not become pregnant. For ease of interpretation, it is best to choose an age value at which women can actually become pregnant. If we choose the value 0, then the interpretation and estimate of b_2 would not change, but $\exp(b_1)$ would be the odds ratio for breast cancer for women who became pregnant at the age of zero versus women who never became pregnant. The odds ratio for the third woman compared to the first would become $\exp(b_1 + b_2 \times 35)$. The interpretation of $\exp(b_3)$ is not affected by the choice.

(d) The only parameter estimates that change value are the ones that refer to the columns **tr.prop4** and **tr.prop6**. They play a similar role as **pregnant**. They become $1.921 + 5 \times 0.019 = 2.016$ and $2.114 + 5 \times 0.019 = 2.209$ respectively. The parameters that give information of the CCR5-Δ32 deletion are not affected.

3. We would create two transition-specific covariables, say `aids.time.4` and `aids.time.6`. In `aids.time.4`, the value `11.46` in the last row of `aids.time` becomes zero. In `aids.time.6`, the other two non-zero values in `aids.time` become zero.

4. (a) Before 1997, the effect of HCV coinfection on liver related mortality was $\exp(3.48)$. The effect after 1997 was $\exp(3.48 - 1.17)$, hence a factor $\exp(-1.17)$ lower.

(b) The *additional* change in AIDS-specific hazard in IDU, compared to the MSM group, if we compare the cART period to the pre-cART period, is assumed to be the same in HIV mono-infected and coinfected IDUs.

In the answers, β_k refers to the parameter in row number k.

(c) We need to compare HCV coinfected IDU with HIV mono-infected IDU. The parameters are read from column 5. The relative hazard is $\exp(\beta_1 + \beta_{21}) = \exp(3.48 + 0.26) = 42$.

(d) Now we look at column 13, and compare this with column 9. There is one extra term, which is quantified by β_8. The relative hazard becomes $\exp(3.48 - 1.17 + 0.26) = \exp(3.74) = 13$.

(e) We look at the relevant terms in column 6 that refer to male IDUs aged 30 that do not occur in column 2. Since we compare *within* the IDU group, the parameter β_{16} for the IDU group relative to MSM cancels. The relative hazard is $\exp(\beta_2 + \beta_{16} + \beta_{21} - \beta_{16}) = \exp(\beta_2 + \beta_{21}) = \exp(-0.19) = 0.83$.

(f) We need to compare HCV coinfected female MSW with HIV mono-infected female MSW. The effect is found by adding the cells in column 14 that apply to HCV coinfected female MSW and subtracting the ones in column 10 that apply to HIV mono-infected female MSW. We obtain $\exp(\beta_2 + \beta_9 + \beta_{15}) = \exp(1.19) = 3.29$.

(g) There is an additional effect of age, parameter β_{25}. Hence we have $\exp(1.19 + 0.09) = 3.6$. Note that the age effect is given per 10 years increase.

(h) For both groups, the parameters are read from column 10. The parameters β_{16} and β_{19} give the additional effect of IDUs. The relative hazard is $\exp(\beta_{16} + \beta_{19}) = \exp(0.66) = 1.93$.

(i) For both groups, the parameters are read from column 14. The parameters that are specific for IDU are β_{16}, β_{19} and β_{21}. The parameter β_{15} is specific for MSW. The relative hazard is $\exp(\beta_{16} + \beta_{19} + \beta_{21} - \beta_{15}) = \exp(0.76) = 2.14$.

(j) The effect is found by adding the cells in column 14 that apply to HCV coinfected male IDU and subtracting the ones in column 6 that apply to HCV coinfected male IDU. The relative hazard is $\exp(\beta_5 + \beta_9 + \beta_{19}) = \exp(-1.3) = 0.27$.

Chapter 5: Regression; Translation to Cumulative Scale

1. We use the relation

$$F_k(t) = \int_0^t \lambda_k(s)\overline{F}(s)ds$$

$\overline{F}(s)$ can be written as $\exp\{-[\Lambda_1(s) + \Lambda_2(s)]\}$. Λ_1 is the same in both groups, but $\Lambda_2(s|I) > \Lambda_2(s|II)$. Therefore, $\overline{F}(s|I) < \overline{F}(s|II)$, which implies $F_1(t|I) < F_2(t|I)$. By the one-to-one relation between cause-specific cumulative incidence and subdistribution hazard, we derive that the subdistribution hazard for cause 1 is smaller in group I.

2. The statement is not correct. $\Lambda_{\text{AIDS}}(t \mid \text{ccr5}_i)$ and $\Lambda_{\text{SI}}(t \mid \text{ccr5}_i)$ are the cumulative cause-specific hazards. They are equal to the marginal cumulative hazards for AIDS and SI if and only if time to AIDS and time to SI are independent. Only in that case the relation defines independence. Otherwise, the product structure holds, but only for the cause-specific hazard.

Chapter 6: Epilogue

1. A switch to SI does not prevent AIDS to occur. This is different from an event like pre-AIDS mortality. When we describe and estimate the marginal hazard of AIDS, we ignore the possible switch to SI phenotype.

2. The curves estimate the overall cumulative event probability, with AIDS and pre-AIDS death combined. They can only be interpreted as estimates of the marginal distribution of time to AIDS if all individuals that died before AIDS would have developed AIDS immediately afterwards. This is unlikely to be the case.

3. The cause-specific hazard is often interpeted as marginal hazard. Sometimes this happens because of plain ignorance, sometimes it is deliberately chosen as surrogate measure. However, we have seen that it is not always

justified and marginal hazard ratios may be different (see the example of time to AIDS in IDUs).

In general, marginal hazard and subdistribution hazard are different concepts. If the competing events are independent, regression on the subdistribution hazard has no relation to regression on the marginal hazard. They are equal only if individuals that experience the competing risk would never have experienced the event of interest, as is the case when such individuals are "cured" for the event of interest. ,

The statement is an adapted version of one made in [95, p.460].

4. Probably not. There may be informative censoring, namely when individuals die of AIDS without ever having had KS. Those that are not infected by the human herpesvirus 8 (HHV8) do not develop KS. Hence, their time to death and their potential time to KS are negatively correlated. Other persons died before they developed KS, but were more likely to develop KS had they remained alive than the individuals that did not die and remained in follow-up. In these individuals, time to death and time to KS are positively correlated.

In fact, the marginal hazard, although it can be formulated as theoretical concept, is hard to interpret. It describes the rate of Kaposi's sarcoma that would be observed after HIV infection if mortality due to other AIDS defining illnesses were eliminated. A setting in which the other AIDS defining illnesses do not occur at all is completely hypothetical.

An alternative is to consider all AIDS events in the analysis, for example via a multi-state model. In this way, it can be investigated whether the occurrence of AIDS events after the index diagnosis accelerates progression to death.

5. Since they address "potential bias", the purpose of their study seems to be the causal effect of β-blockers. Such an effect is better quantified by the cause-specific hazard. It may be that the lower subdistribution hazard for PCa-specific mortality in individuals that use β-blockers is completely explained by the fact that they have higher cardiac mortality. If individuals live shorter, prostate cancer is less likely to develop, but this does not necessarily imply a causal effect. A similar argument against their use of the Fine and Gray model was given in [14].

6. There is no guarantee that it is a valid explanation. A model for the subdistribution hazard was used. Let's simplify the setting and assume that treatment failure and treatment interruption are the only two competing events. If the ones who interrupt treatment are less likely to fail, the most extreme scenario occurs when they will never fail. Then the marginal hazard would be the same as the subdistribution hazard and the marginal hazard ratio would be equal to the reported one.

It could be a possible explanation if the observed hazard ratios were from a model for the cause-specific hazard. If the individuals that interrupt treatment are less likely to fail, they would remain in the risk set for a longer period if they had not interrupted. Since a higher percentage interrupts in the early starters, it concerns a larger fraction and thus has a bigger impact. If we again consider the extreme situation that individuals that interrupt treatment would never fail, then the marginal hazard equals the subdistribution hazard and we can refer to Exercise 5.6.1: a larger interruption-specific hazard in early starters and equal failure-specific hazards in both groups implies a smaller subdistribution hazard for failure in the early starters, hence a smaller marginal hazard.

Index

Aalen-Johansen, *see* nonparametric estimator
acyclic, *see* multi-state analysis, irreversible model
alternate format, *see* display formats
at risk, 29

calendar time scale, *see* time, calendar scale
censoring
    administrative, 9, 22, 42, 68, 75, 92
    artificial, 9
    competing risks, 9, 23
    informative, 16–18, 20–24, 63
    interval, 10, 87, 125
    left, 10, 12, 105
    loss to follow-up, 9, 23
    right, 8, 29
    state dependent, 112
censoring complete information, *see* censoring, administrative
clock forward approach, *see* time, clock forward
clock reset approach, *see* time, clock reset
competing risks analysis
    censored data, 17
    multi-state approach, 60–62, 79
    subdistribution approach, 62–63, 80
    when?, 14, 24–27, 213–216
continuous distribution, *see* time, continuous
copula, 21
counting process, 40, 192
covariable, 30

compound, 148
time-varying, 12, 27, 38, 39, 41–43, 164, 184, 192–195
type-specific, 149, 159
covariable, external, *see* covariable, time-varying
covariable, internal, *see* covariable, time-varying
covariable, transition-specific, *see* covariable, type-specific
covariate, *see* covariable
Cox model, *see* proportional hazards
crude risk, *see* cumulative incidence, cause-specific
cumulative incidence, 13
    cause-specific, 14, 29, 60–63
    marginal, 14
    overall, 14, 61, 64
cure model, 88, 194

data format
    stacked long, 111, 146, 157
    state-ordered wide, 111, 116
    time-ordered wide, 111
    transition-based long, 111, 117
delayed entry, *see* left truncation
dependent censoring, *see* censoring, informative
directed graph, 107
discrete distribution, *see* time, discrete
display formats, 66

empirical cumulative distribution function, *see* nonparametric estimator
etiology, 2, 105, 213–216

Printed and bound by CPI Group (UK) Ltd, Croydon, CR0 4YY

23/10/2024

01777673-0007